AN INTRODUCTION

TO

POSITIVE LONGEVITY

HOW TO LIVE BETTER FOR LONGER

TABLE OF CONTENTS

ABSTRACT

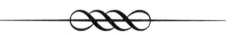

My name is Alexandre and I have spent my life in pursuit of a healthier lifestyle. As a child, I was overweight and pre-diabetic, but despite this, I always had an interest in healthy living. Through trial and error, experimentation with different diets and exercise regimens, as well as an overall commitment to wellness, I was able to not only overcome obesity but also manage eating disorders that had plagued me for years.

In this book on longevity based on my life experience and extensive research, I will share the wisdom and knowledge gained through my journey towards better health. You'll discover scientific researches, practical tips for improving your diet and fitness habits; learn how to make lasting changes to your lifestyle; understand the importance of stress management; explore the connection between physical health and mental wellbeing; gain insight into managing chronic illnesses like diabetes or heart disease; plus so much more! It's time to take control of your own health destiny - let's get started!

According to an increasing number of studies during the past ten years, aging is accompanied by progressive alterations to epigenetic information in both dividing and non-dividing studies.

Epigenetic modifications appear to significantly impact the aging process, according to functional investigations in model organisms and humans.

Drawing on these studies, several notable conclusions could be made - the most prominent of which are as follows.: our life span is largely epigenetically determined rather than genetically predetermined; diet and other environmental factors can affect our life span by altering the epigenetic information, and inhibitors of epigenetic enzymes can affect the life span of model organisms.

Recent findings have illuminated the biological processes driving aging, providing newfound insight into this universal phenomenon. Enabling us to comprehend the processes at work in aging and how they influence our bodies.

Subsequently, these findings uncover immense opportunities for therapeutic treatment of aging and age-related diseases like cancer thanks to the reversibility of epigenetic information.

INTRODUCTION

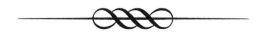

A ll living things experience aging, a complex multifactorial biological process, which can be defined as a time-dependent, progressive reduction in typical physiological activities.

Despite having the same amount of DNA, environmental factors, like nutrition, cause distinct changes to the stored epigenetic information, which lead to a noticeable difference in the physical characteristics, reproductive habits, and lifespan of the queen and worker honeybees. Transcriptional drift and genomic instability result from the ensuing variation in the pattern of epigenetic information within individual cells in the population as we age. Epigenetic information is established by enzymes and is reversible. Therefore, unlike genetic alterations, which are currently theoretically irreversible in humans, epigenetics holds considerable promise for therapeutic intervention targeting. As a result, defining and comprehending the epigenetic changes that occur as we age is a significant field of ongoing research that has the potential to change humanity.

Werner syndrome and Hutchinson-Gilford progeria syndrome are rare genetic conditions that cause accelerated aging traits, as well as premature mortality. These illnesses can be utilized to gain a better understanding of the biological processes involved in human aging due to their resemblance with natural physiological maturing. A mutation in the DNA repair mechanism is to blame for these disorders, resulting in disordered structure in the way chromosomes are built. The causal mutations of these syndromes indicate that chromatin breakdown and genomic instability are important elements in human aging. Furthermore, by comprehending the molecular pathophysiology of these human disorders of accelerated aging, we are better able to understand the intricate aging process. Unlike individuals who age with typical aging symptoms, those living with HGPS experience a segmental progeria that affects isolated tissues; thus they do not display the same effects as seen in normal aging. These models give us a unique chance to comprehend the aging process in a human model by replicating some molecular and cellular alterations that are traits of the natural aging process.

According to studies in humans and these potent aging models, the epigenome experiences a progressive loss in its configuration during aging, just like all other biological structures inside the cells. The chromosomal architecture, genomic integrity, and gene expression patterns are significantly altered. Where studied, these effects are mainly constant from simple single-celled eukaryotes like budding yeast to sophisticated multicellular ones. We can see the aging process more clearly thanks to these conserved processes. Here, we will go over the epigenetic modifications that have recently been found to substantially impact the aging process, from research on single-celled model organisms to human aging models. We will summarize the most recent advancements in this field and identify future possibilities for the future.

After sexual maturity, there is a steady loss of molecular fidelity known as aging, which leads to function loss, disease, and eventually death. The rate of aging is inversely correlated with the mean lifespan in most animals. Additionally, aging is the most significant risk factor for cardiovascular disease, cancer, and neurodegeneration. Conversely, the length of time an organism is free from chronic sickness is referred to as its "health span." One of the fascinating topics of biogerontology study is how to extend lifespan and health span.

Various animal models have been essential for identifying critical aging-related mechanisms. Researchers have studied replicative lifespans, determined by the maximum number of mitotic divisions a cell can go through, and chronological lifespan, determined by the amount of time a cell can survive in a post-mitotic state, using genetically tractable models such as yeast. In addition, the short lifespans of worms and flies have been used as a research tool in other investigations. Although studies using these models have made significant contributions to the field, they fall short of adequately capturing the complexity of human aging, especially in light of age-related disorders and the shortening of health spans. So, using the genetic similarity to humans and the availability of gene knockout and premature aging models, vertebrate models such as mice have been used. The African turquoise killifish, which lives for 4-6 months and mimics many of the age-related pathological changes found in humans, is a suitable alternative short-lived vertebrate model because, unfortunately, mouse lifespan is too long for adequate laboratory studies of normal aging.

Studies using different models have shown that genetic variations and somatic mutations are the causes of longevity. However, non-genetic factors also play a significant role. For example, restricting calories decreases basal metabolic rate, increases stress response, and restores the balance of mitonuclear proteins. In addition, reduced fertility is related to an increase in lifespan. These findings shed light on how "epi"-genetic factors affect longevity pathways.

CHAPTER 1

LIVING LONGER AND BETTER

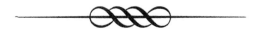

With this Special Health tips, you will discover the preventative measures experts advise for keeping your mind and body in shape for an active and fulfilling life. Maintaining good vision, hearing, and memory and receiving retentiveness, strengthen your bones, reduce joint pain, and lower your risk of heart disease. Additionally, you will receive expert advice to help maximize your health care budget, choose a health plan that suits your needs, and create a health care proxy.

Make the most of your time now to read this tips updated health, wellbeing, and planning guide.

10 Ways to Live Longer and Better

Something extraordinary is taking place. Not just a little bit longer, but much longer; we live longer lives than at any other time in history. The typical American's life expectancy was around 46 years in 1900; today, it is getting close to 80. The typical life expectancy is that. Many of us live to be over 80 or even 100 years old!

It's good that so many of us are living longer. However, as people age, diseases like arthritis, hip fractures, memory loss, etc., become more likely. It's critical to realize that these symptoms aren't a typical aspect of aging. They are more likely to appear as we age, but aging should not be viewed as a given for their development.

The excellent thing is that we have considerable control over how quickly we age., including how quickly and, perhaps more significantly, how well. Nobody always appears their age. Some 60-year-olds appear to be 40, while others look 60. How come?

Aging is influenced by three factors: genetics, environment, and lifestyle. While the people who gave us our DNA cannot be changed, we can pick our environment and way of life. The last two elements have a significant impact on how well we age.

In light of this, the following ten suggestions will help you live longer and have a higher quality lifestyle:

1. Manage your tension:

Stress, especially persistent stress, ages us more quickly than a few other things. For example, ever notice how presidents deteriorate so quickly when in office? We all stress our lives, which could even be beneficial in moderation. However, stress starts to impact when it becomes a regular part of our lives. Even though we can't completely get rid of stress, there are things we can do to lessen it.

2. Keep your blood pressure in check:

In contemporary society, hypertension is a very frequent issue. Your body can suffer physical harm from high blood pressure, which also puts you at higher risk for vascular disease and stroke. Consider your blood's flow throughout your body as the plumbing in your home. When water pressure increases to the point that it can burst a pipe, that is the equivalent of a stroke in your body. If it stays high all the time, it will subject the pipes to unnecessary wear and tear, reducing their lifespan, which is analogous to Your body's arteries stiffening due to atherosclerosis. the excellent thing is that high blood pressure can be controlled with correct diagnosis and management. It's crucial to monitor your blood pressure frequently and maintain good control over it. A healthy, low-salt diet, exercise, and diet can all be helpful.

3. Quit smoking:

This practically goes without saying. Smoking, as we all know, greatly increases the chance of heart and lung disease. But did you know that it also quickens aging, especially regarding the skin? It will, without a doubt, shorten your life and perhaps the lives of those who breathe in the secondhand smoke around you. Don't criticize yourself if you smoke and have tried unsuccessfully to stop. The decision to stop smoking is among the most difficult. Keep trying, then. Most successful people need numerous tries to succeed. According to Mark Twain, one of the simplest things to do is stop smoking. Since I've done it a thousand times, I should know.

4. Get some shut-eye:

Okay, get up. This is quite significant. One of the most overlooked factors of health may be sleep. Why is sleep necessary? In many respects, sleep is still a mystery to science. However, recent research has revealed its significant impact on general health. Its significance for preserving a healthy memory, something many of us worry about as we age, makes it even more fascinating. Sleep aids in helping the information we learn during the day stick in our brains, as is now well established. How much sleep do we therefore need? Every night, at least seven to eight hours.

Many of us find it difficult, but that should always be our objective. Sleep is crucial for more than simply memory. Lack of sleep can raise blood pressure, lead to sadness, and decrease lifespan if it becomes a way of life. Eliminating caffeine in the late afternoon and at night is a helpful sleep-related suggestion. However, after ingesting caffeine, it remains in our bodies for several hours. Therefore, cut off or switch to decaf that final cup of coffee after dinner.

5. Continue to eat healthfully:

Most of us are aware of which foods are healthy and unhealthful. The best nutrition advice is to avoid depriving yourself of meals you enjoy to shed pounds or stay healthy. One of life's fundamental pleasures is eating. Eat the foods you enjoy, but watch your portion sizes. The most important thing is to eat a diversified diet with lots of fruits and vegetables. Most of us frequently consume the same foods. Sincerely, do you not always put the same items in your cart when you go grocery shopping? Be courageous. Now and then, try something different. A diversified diet is healthful.

6. Work out your physique:

Move. Simply move. Utilizing your muscles and bones is necessary to maintain your youth. Find a hobby you like to do. If you don't like what you're doing, you won't stick with it. Don't run on a treadmill if you detest it. Play tennis if you enjoy it. Commit to doing it frequently, even if it's only a simple stroll. Move.

7. Challenge your mind:

Your mind is incredible; it is who you are. It gives you identity. Your brain stores all of your memories and feelings; it also allows you to laugh, grieve, create, appreciate art and music, and even experience love. You should make every effort to maintain a young, healthy brain. In addition to the other suggestions, using your brain regularly is the greatest way to maintain it. Keep learning new things to keep your mind active. Replace the mundane with something new. Look for novel encounters. Learning and challenges are what your brain thrives on. Be a student throughout your life.

8. Remain upbeat:

"The more I see me; I'll be," goes the proverb. If you decide to perceive yourself as old and incapable, you'll probably act and behave accordingly. The operative verb is "select."You have a choice in how you see the world and yourself. Even situations beyond your control can be positively controlled with the right mindset. Getting furious or angry will not make the traffic move if you are stuck in it. Instead, you can decide to accept the situation while you reflect, pray, or listen to music. You won't stay young and healthy if you let stress consume you and raise your blood pressure.

9. Uphold intimate connections:

Beyond just being painful emotionally, loneliness and solitude are harmful to our health. It is crucial to have people in our lives. Naturally, things change as we get older – kids move away, friends pass away. But we can venture out and make new friends. Continue to engage with others. Go to lessons. Volunteer. Invite someone to a new restaurant for dinner. Even acquiring a pet, Studies have demonstrated that social interaction makes people live longer and in better health. I told my father many years ago that married people live longer than single individuals. He made the amusing comment that getting married doesn't make you live longer; it simply makes it look that way.

10. be religious:

Pascal, a philosopher from the 17th century, reportedly said: "Man's incapacity to remain quietly in a room alone is the root of all humanity's troubles." More than ever, our body, mind, and spirit require periods of quiet reflection and serenity. It might be a quiet time for reflection or prayer. Such moments have a lot of power, which shouldn't be understated. They facilitate clarity, comfort, and peace in our hectic life.

Therefore, it appears that we may all anticipate living a lot longer. Why not make the most of that time with the intention of quality and health? It's your decision whether or not to live a long and fulfilling life.

CHAPTER 2

HOW IS LONGEVITY DEFINED?

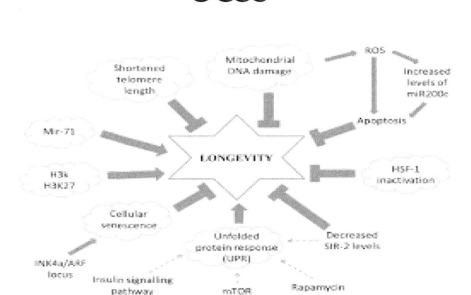

Longevity is frequently defined by biologists as the typical lifespan anticipated under ideal circumstances. However, it's challenging to define the ideal. Therefore, numerous studies in medicine are being done to determine the "correct" kind and amount of exercise you should do, the ideal diet to follow, and whether or not specific medications or dietary supplements can lengthen your life.

Considerable increase in life expectancy, in part due to medical breakthroughs that have practically totally eradicated some dangerous infectious diseases.

A neonate born in 1900 had a 50-year lifespan on average. In the United States, the average life expectancy is currently close to 79 years— 81 years for women and 76 years for men1—and it is considerably longer in certain other countries.

Humans will likely live far longer than we currently think. People may live longer if people can establish the optimum circumstances of a good diet and exercise.

"Long life" or "a great duration of life" are definitions of longevity. The word is derived from the Latin longevity. So you can see how the concepts of longus (long) and aevum (age) are combined to imply someone who lives a long period in this term.

The comparative character of this definition is its most crucial component. Long life means that something is more extended than something, and the average lifetime is that something.

How You Can Increase Your Longevity

A person is said to have longevity if they live longer than the typical individual. Longevity is the pursuit of your highest potential age. By putting healthy habits and attitudes into practice, this may be possible to achieve.

What Affects How Long You Live?

You might believe that your genes control how long you live, but genetics only contribute up to 30% of life expectancy. Your actions, attitudes, surroundings, and a small amount of luck account for the remaining factors.

Various methods for extending your life may have been mentioned to you. Remember that none have been demonstrated in humans, and the majority are merely theories. Living a healthy lifestyle is the only way to extend your life.

CHAPTER 3

HOW TO INCREASE
YOUR LIFESPAN

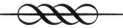

What should you do to maximize your longevity and surpass the average? Here is a list of factors to think about:

1. **Regular exercise:** According to research, regular moderate exercise can turn back theclock on your DNA.

2. **Put plenty of vegetables on your plate:** Almost every diet believes that eating moreveggies is the way to go, despite many disagreements over the ideal diet for extending a lifetime.

3. **Take into account sporadic fasting (with many variations on how this is achieved):** It has been demonstrated that fasting considerably increases mice's lifespan (and health). In addition, caloric restriction increases the lifespan of test species like mice, according to research from the 1930s. In a 2018 study that was published in Cell Metabolism, 53 non- obese adult humans were followed for

two years. The test group cut back on calories by 15%. In addition, according to metabolic investigations, the test group exhibited more minor oxidative stress/damage than the control group.

4. **Get adequate sleep:** Most people function at their best after a night of seven to nine hours of sleep. Take care to control your tension. Stress can negatively impact your body andencourage negative habits like smoking or binge eating.

5. **Foster close connections with others:** Spending time with our loved ones increases longevity, possibly because it reduces stress or dangerous behaviors. Researchers at the University of Exeter Medical School in England found that volunteers had a death rate that was22% lower than non-volunteers in one trial.

Is longevity determined by genetics?

What is genetic?

Genetics is the branch of biology concerned with the study of the DNA of organisms, how their DNA manifests as genes, and how those genes are inherited by offspring. Genes are passed to offspring in both sexual and asexual reproduction, and over time natural selection can accumulate variations amongst individuals on the group level, in the process known as evolution.

Genetics, environment, and lifestyle all impact how long people live. With significant food and clean water availability, better housing and living circumstances decreased exposure to infectious diseases, and more access to medical treatment, environmental changes starting in the 1900s dramatically increased the average life duration. The public health advancements that lowered newborn mortality raised the likelihood that children would survive childhood and prevented infection and communicable diseases were the most significant. As a result, the average lifespan in the United States is around 80 years, while some people live significantly longer.

Scientists are researching persons in their 90s (known as nonagenarians) and 100s (known as centenarians, including supercentenarians, ages 110+) to see what factors contribute to their long lives. They discovered that people who live long lives differ significantly in terms of occupation, money, and education. The differences they do have, however, reflect their lifestyles; many are stress-tolerant, nonsmokers, and do not have obesity. Moreover, most are female. As a result, these older persons are less prone than their counterparts of the same age to develop age-related chronic diseases, such as high blood pressure, heart disease, cancer, and diabetes, due to their healthy lifestyle choices.

First-degree relatives are those who have a first-degree relative with a long-lived person. These persons are more likely to live longer and in better health than their peers. At age 70, the age- related illnesses prevalent in older persons are less likely to affect people whose parents are centenarians. The siblings of centenarians frequently enjoy long lives, and if they develop age- related illnesses (such as high blood pressure, heart disease, cancer, or type 2 diabetes), these illnesses manifest later than they do in the general population. The tendency for longer lifespans to run in families raises the possibility that shared genetics, lifestyle choices, or both significantly impact longevity.

Genes associated with long life are now being studied. About 25% of the diversity in human life expectancy is thought to be genetically determined. However, it is unclear which genes and how they affect longevity. The APOE, FOXO3, and CETP genes have a few common changes (referred to as polymorphisms) related to extended life lengths, although they are not present in all people with remarkable longevity. It's possible that several different genes, some of which have undiscovered variations, work together to promote long life.

The same gene variations that raise disease risk in humans with ordinary life spans have been found in supercentenarians through whole-genome sequencing research. But other newly discovered gene variants in the supercentenarians might favor lifespan. There has been a noticeable increase in life expectancy over the years, partly due to medical improvements that have virtually eradicated some major infectious diseases. Some people can achieve a healthy old age with nutritious eating, moderate alcohol use, quitting smoking, and regular exercise; genetics then appear to play an increasingly significant part in maintaining individuals' health as they age into their eighties and beyond. On the other hand, many nonagenarians and centenarians can live independently and stay healthy well into their later years.

Some gene variations that support a long life are connected to the fundamental upkeep and operation of the body's cells. These biological processes include DNA repair, maintenance of the telomere sections at the ends of chromosomes, and defense of cells against injury by unstable oxygen-containing molecules (free radicals). In addition, the risk of heart disease (the leading cause of mortality in older adults), stroke, and insulin resistance is considerably decreased by other genes linked to blood fat (lipid) levels, inflammation, and the cardiovascular and immune systems.

In addition to researching the elderly in the United States, researchers are also looking at a few places throughout the globe where individuals regularly survive above the age of 90, including Sardinia, Okinawa, and Ikaria in Greece (Italy). These three regions are comparable because they have lower income levels, less industrialization, and a propensity for traditional (non- Western) lifestyles. They are also similar in that they are somewhat separated from the rest of their countries' populations. For example, in Sardinia, a sizable part of the very old is men, in contrast to other people, the elderly. Scientists are examining whether hormones, sex-specific genes, or other elements may affect both men and women living longer lives on this island.

CHAPTER 4

HUMAN LONGEVITY:
GENETICS OR LIFESTYLE?

A fortunate fusion of hereditary and non-genetic variables controls healthy aging and longevity in humans. According to family research, genetic variables account for around 25% of the variation in human longevity. The critical genetic variables influencing the individual variance of the aging phenotype have been identified as genes associated with cell maintenance and its fundamental metabolism through investigating the genetic and molecular foundation of aging. A low-calorie diet and/or a genetically efficient metabolism of nutrients can modulate lifespan by supporting effective cell and organism maintenance, according to studies on calorie restriction and the diversity of genes linked to nutrient-sensing signaling. Recent epigenetic research has demonstrated that epigenetic changes, which are influenced by both genetic make-up and lifestyle choices, are very responsive to the aging process and can either be a biomarker of the quality of aging or affect the rate and quality of aging.

Overall, research has demonstrated the importance of treatments that control how genetic background and environment interact to affect an individual's likelihood of living a long life.

Due to the social and medical burden associated with the continuous increase in lifespan in western countries and the resulting growth in the elderly population, research on aging, and in particular the search for the factors that contribute to successful aging and longevity, has been steadily expanding over the past few decades. The relationship between genetic make-up and lifestyle in determining a person's likelihood of delaying aging (perhaps without age-related diseases and disabilities) and longevity is one of the significant problems in this discipline. It was possible to better grasp this association thanks to the data gained by bio gerontologists in recent years, which identified most of the molecular and biochemical pathways involved in aging. This has led to the development of crucial techniques centered on potential lifestyle treatments to enhance longevity by modifying the fundamental biological pathways of aging.

Aging's genetic component

The notion that aging is inevitable and unaffected by genetics was widely held before the 1990ies. The idea that aging happens after reproduction and that there is no longer a requirement for selection to act on genes expressed during this late stage of life was crucial in this perspective.

When you're not at your healthiest, you can probably tell. You may simply feel "off." You may find that you feel tired, your digestive system isn't functioning as well as it normally does, and you seem to catch colds. Mentally, you may find you can't concentrate and feel anxious or depressed.

The good news: a healthy lifestyle can help you feel better. Even better, you don't have to overhaul your entire life overnight. It's pretty easy to make a couple of small changes that can steer you in the direction of improved well-being. And once you make one change, that success can motivate you to continue to make more positive shifts.

CHAPTER 5

WHAT IS A "HEALTHY LIFESTYLE"?

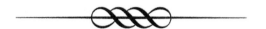

C hoosing and putting into practice habits that would improve one's health as part of daily planning requires managing all behavior that might impact one's health. Healthy lifestyle choices are those that uphold and improve an individual's degree of health. These behaviors include maintaining a sufficient and balanced diet, managing stress, getting regular exercise, realizing one's potential spiritually, forming supportive relationships with others, and taking charge of one's health. The choice and organization of meals and the person's values in terms of food are all aspects of an adequate and balanced diet.

The ability to identify and utilize one's physiological and psychological resources to lessen or effectively control the stress one experiences is referred to as stress management. The regular physical activity entails specific low-intensity, moderate-intensity, and high-intensity physical activities. Internal resource development is a key component of spiritual progress. The individual working towards their life goals maximizes their power regarding their wellness status. Therefore, this feature as self-actualization in their studies.

The individual's ties with others are considered in interpersonal relations and support. The need to safeguard and enhance health refers to the person's active sense of accountability for their well-being.

Studies show that leading a healthy lifestyle can help prevent many adult illnesses. The most common causes of death are cancer, diabetes, heart disease, and persistent respiratory problems. Similar findings were made in the National Disease Burden 2004 survey, which discovered that cardiovascular diseases in Turkey are to blame for 43% of male fatalities and 52% of female fatalities. According to studies, there is a relatively small list of risk factors for chronic diseases, including smoking, eating poorly, being inactive, drinking alcohol, having uncontrollably high blood pressure, and having high body fat percentages. Only 5-10% of cancer cases are genetically predisposed, with environmental factors and lifestyle decisions being the main contributors. The study's findings highlighted that many adult ailments, including heart attacks, paralysis, chronic respiratory conditions, and cancer, may be avoided by adopting good lifestyle choices from infancy.

A variety of learned skills are required for healthy living. Teaching the skills needed for healthy living heavily relies on the wellness idea and its models.

Wellness

In psychology, counseling, and medicine, the idea of well-being has become more prevalent. In a study where they analyzed several studies on wellness in medical literature, it was found that although previous studies were primarily undertaken to define wellness, more current studies have gone beyond that. In reality, the idea of wellness is now used in the execution of health programs and as a strategy for improving health. In addition, wellness has developed into a concept that is used in all sectors of the healthcare industry. Studies link this phrase to several other ideas that they consider to be related.

Assert that while the ideas of wellness and psychological well-being, health, and life quality share some characteristics, they also have some distinctive properties. Wellness is holistic and multifaceted; it emphasizes healthy lifestyle choices, is connected to activities or processes, and looks at how people and their environments interact.

Have also looked at the literature's definitions of wellness. They consequently discovered that wellness is seen in these definitions as a decision, a method, and a way of life. Additionally, they found that, although multi-factorial, well-being exhibits a holistic framework and is subjective and relative. It emphasizes balance and displays the qualities of healthy individuals.

Although "wellness" has several definitions, the most popular one is that it refers to a person's overall habits focused on maintaining optimal health. These actions include working toward one's objectives and those for a more meaningful existence, integrating one's body, mind, and spirit, and leading a productive life in all social, personal, and ecological spheres. These justifications highlight the fact that well-being is a way of life. In an attempt to describe wellness, various models have been constructed in the literature, as was mentioned earlier. The Wheel of Wellness Model was established and is one of the most researched wellness models. Our nation has also seen articles about this model. Following these investigations, this model changed its structure and content, becoming The Indivisible Self: An Evidence-Based Model of Wellness. Despite not being called the "indivisible self" like previous models, this one exhibits a multi-factorial structure.

These five aspects are the physical self, the social self, the creative self, the coping self, and the fundamental self.

A different model was created. Physical, emotional, social, mental, spiritual, and environmental elements are subfactors.

The Well-Star Scale Model (WSSM), a five-factor model that takes advantage of factors highlighted in most models in the literature, was developed in Turkey using the star metaphor. In a later study, these elements are identified as emotional, life purpose and goal-orientation, cognitive, social, and physical components. For example, realizing one's feelings, managing them, and taking care of themselves, for their life situations, and any disputes in a realistic, positive, and constructive way are all qualities of emotional wellness. Meaning of life and goal-orientedness Wellness involves qualities like looking for the meaning of life, choosing a goal, and working toward it. The cognitive wellness factor involves traits like enjoying being intellectually active, being open to learning, and problem-solving. Social wellness shows the quality and degree of individuals' interactions with others. In addition, this factor involves the social support perceived by people who are important in the individual's life. Physical wellness involves elements related to a healthy lifestyle, generally implementing physical health-oriented behaviors such as having balanced and adequate dietary habits and maintaining a physically active life.

These models serve an instructive function as they point to which niches need examination when working with an advisee. When carrying out psychological services, these models facilitate the efforts of psychological counselors and other mental health professionals. The article by Myers et al. (2000) plays a highly instructive role in this subject.

Healthy Lifestyle Behaviors and Wellness

Stating that there is confusion about the connection between the concepts of wellness and health, Greenberg (1985) argues that health is a conceptualization of social, cognitive, emotional, spiritual, and physical elements and asserts that, conceptually, wellness is a consolidation of these elements. High-level wellness is the state of these elements being in balance. In health-related professions, the state of being healthy is approached in the form of improving, protecting, and maintaining health. To actualize this, individuals need to maintain their healthy lifestyle behaviors and that these behaviors are features that maintain and raise the wellness levels of individuals.

The literature shows that wellness is viewed as a healthy lifestyle. Additionally, indicate that a healthy lifestyle reduces the risk of contracting certain diseases and increases wellness; therefore, a healthy lifestyle affects health and wellness. According to them, even though factors not directly controlled by individuals—such as environmental factors like air pollution, hereditary factors, and factors like an inadequate healthcare system-affect their health and wellness, their healthy living habits can still prevent some diseases. However, studies on the relationship between wellness and healthy lifestyles appear to be limited in the literature. For that purpose, as a result of a study done, it was determined that a major 68% of total wellness could be explained via dietary habits, spiritual growth, and interpersonal relationships. Also, in analyses related to the subfactors of wellness, it was found that some healthy lifestyle behaviors predict the subfactors of wellness. In short, according to studies, there is a close relationship between a healthy lifestyle and the wellness of an individual.

In this part, different developmental periods were discussed in the three groups.

These groups are the childhood-adolescence period, the university student/emerging adulthood period, and the adulthood/advanced age period.

Childhood-Adolescence Period and Wellness

It is stated that no group is as important as children and young people in the learning and adoption of healthy behaviors and healthy lifestyle choices.

This is because most healthy or unhealthy habits are learned in childhood and adolescence and are often hard to change. In a qualitative study examining the wellness of children, it is stressed that the caregivers responsible for the child's care are important for the child's healthy lifestyle. It was seen that even though the caregivers had the role of giving care to the child, they did not adopt the role of conveying a healthy lifestyle. However, it is not only the caregivers but also the environment in which they are present that is important for the wellness of children. In this regard, it has been proven that wellness-based prevention programs in schools involving body image, personal attitude, and eating behaviors are effective. In certain states in America (e.g., Colorado), the implementation of wellness policies is mandatory in schools. A qualitative study of 25 young Americans in the emerging adulthood period determined that childhood experiences influence emotional, physical, and spiritual wellness. All kinds of practices related to healthy lifestyles, such as healthy eating habits and physical activities at school and home, affect wellness in emotional, physical, and spiritual aspects in different ways. A meta study examining over weighted /obesity in children emphasized the importance of increasing life quality and mental health through wellness.

Most lifestyle choices are acquired during the period of adolescence. However, unhealthy habits and lifestyles chosen during this period can lead to certain physical and emotional diseases in later years. There are opinions and studies on how some early deaths in adulthood can be mitigated by encouraging healthy habits during adolescence (National

Center for Health Statistics 2000). Because of this, it is advantageous to start teaching young children and teenagers about tangible ways they can live better lifestyles and increase their wellness. Particularly if the habits of maintaining a healthy diet and engaging in physical activity are formed from childhood, these behaviors survive into adolescence.

In the literature, we may encounter studies about the wellness of adolescents. Additionally, when we examine studies conducted with young people, some studies on the concepts of healthy behaviors involved in wellness, subjective well-being, and life satisfaction may be found, even if they may not directly have to do with wellness. Interventions aimed at raising wellness have a positive impact on the academic, emotional, social and physical development of children and young people. Parents, teachers, administrators, psychologists, and psychological counselors are responsible for raising the wellness level of children. A high level of wellness protects adolescents from a series of problems such as substance use. The prevention of problematic behaviors such as substance use, risky sexual behaviors, and violence and the increase of healthy behaviors like a balanced diet and being physically active are important for national health. This is especially true for adolescents. Because these risky behaviors show a tendency to coexist during the adolescence period. There is research that shows that adolescents have risky health behaviors in Turkey. The wellness of adolescents is an important indicator of their future health and lifestyle habits. For this reason, the evaluation of the wellness level of adolescents, especially in the school environment, and the determination of the variables about wellness are viewed to be important for effecting healthy lifestyle behaviors.

In a study conducted with young people ages 12-17 years, it was found that young people at the higher end of the age spectrum have lower wellness scores than others. Other studies also demonstrate this tendency. Similarly, the results of a comparative study on Israeli students' total, creative, essential, and physical wellness display significant differences in favor of the younger students. As we can see, the research indicates that wellness tends to decrease as ages increase during adolescence. The developmental traits brought on by adolescence might concern the explanation of this tendency.

Due to their importance in gaining healthy habits in childhood and adolescence, it is important that the individuals responsible for the education of the children and young people–parents, teachers, mental health professionals, and especially psychological counselors working in schools—be models and conduct activities related to provide wellness improving skills to children and young people. At this point, providing the children with healthy dietary habits from infancy through childhood and taking the necessary precautions for them to maintain these habits at school may play an important role. Thus, various health and social problems that may occur in the future can be prevented. Moreover, providing conditions that support physical activity for students in schools may contribute to raising their wellness level. Especially seeing as how the amount of time that children spend in front of a television or computer screen gradually increases, providing opportunities that enable children to play games involving physical activity and do exercises are thought to be important.

GENERATING HARMONY

Wellness includes striking a balance in our daily lives. A balanced life can mean many different things, depending on the culture, environment, available resources, and other elements. Balance is about making time for the things that bring us joy and fulfillment. This includes engaging in paid or unpaid employment, play, socializing with loved ones, volunteering, engaging in physical activity, including sexual activity, praying, resting, also sleep. What we individually define as "balance" will differ because we all have unique needs, interests, and capacities. And we must occasionally rebalance to respond to the changes in our lives. Balance is crucial when going through a difficult period, whether it be stress, disease, trauma, or an emotional struggle. Our routines and habits might help us regain that sense of control during these challenging moments. We need to emphasize the roles we play in our own lives and the lives of others, including those of students, friends, parents, spouses, churches, hobbyists, community members, and citizens. In defining who we are, what gives us a feeling of purpose, and how our lives are interdependent on other people, animals, and the environment, our roles and connections play a key part. Being actively involved in life and relationships provides a sense of balance and general wellness. For instance, swimming has both physical (increasing circulation and gaining strength) and social (meeting new people), and emotional benefits (relieving stress). However, swimming laps every week is not necessary for health; occasionally, entering the pool is a terrific step. We feel more organized and in control when we live in a clean and safe environment. It offers a chance for couples and families to work together as well as a way to exercise. On the other hand, making time for relaxation might help us achieve balance in our lives. "Downtime" might give us the room we need to consider a problem, process our emotions, or simply relax.

How is it beneficial?

The risk of many diseases, including those that can run in your family, can be decreased by adopting healthy practices.

In a recent study, for instance, persons who ate a typical American diet for 8 weeks—one high in fruits and vegetables—had a lower risk of cardiovascular disease.

In another study, researchers found that every 66-gram increase in daily fruit and vegetable intake resulted in a 25% decrease in the prevalence of type 2 diabetes.

A portion of processed grains can be replaced with whole grains to lower disease risk. In a study of over 200,000 adults, those who consumed whole grains had a type 2 diabetes rate that was 29 percent lower than those who consumed the least.

And a meta-analysis of 45 studies found that consuming 90 grams (or three 30-gram meals) of whole grains daily decreased the risk of cancer by 15%, coronary heart disease by 19%, and cardiovascular disease by 22%.

1. Exercise:

For as little as 11 minutes every day can lengthen your life. Over 44,000 persons were tracked in a 2020 study by academics. The risk of death was decreased in those who exercised for 11 minutes each day compared to those who only did so for 2 minutes. This contrast held even if people spent 8.5 hours each day sitting down.

2. Reduces costs:

It's wise to schedule a yearly physical with your primary care provider. This is particularly relevant because some medical disorders, like high blood pressure, are "silent." As a result, until you are checked, you aren't aware that you have the problem. This implies they don't exhibit any symptoms.

However, the likelihood that you may need to see a doctor decreases as your health improves. In addition, money may be saved by eliminating the need for co-pays, medications, and other treatments.

3. Increases the lifespan:

A longer lifespan is associated with basic healthy behaviors. For example, if you have never smoked, maintained a healthy weight, exercised regularly, drank alcohol in moderation, and ate a balanced diet at 50, you may live up to 14 years longer. If you make even a few changes, your longevity may rise.

4. It could be beneficial to the environment:

Foods that have undergone extreme processing typically include refined grains, flavor, texture, and color enhancers. Cheese puffs, pre-made dessert cakes, chicken nuggets, and sweetened breakfast cereals are a few examples of these items. Foods in American supermarkets are over 70% ultra-processed.

Foods that are extremely processed cause deforestation, water scarcity, a decline in biodiversity, greenhouse gas emissions, and plastic waste.

Then there are items made from animals. According to research by the Food and Agriculture Organization of the United Nations, animals for meat and dairy account for 14.5% of all human-produced greenhouse gases (an organization inside the U.N. that works on eliminating hunger and food inequality globally).

There are quick remedies available, though. Based on the National Resources Defense Council, if every American reduced their weekly beef intake by 1/4 pound, the reduction in greenhouse gas emissions would be the same as removing four to six million cars from the road.

But it's not just a matter of how much or how little you consume. For example, cycling can reduce the quantity of carbon dioxide produced into the atmosphere by taking the place of brief motor trips.

According to a 2010 study that wasn't peer-reviewed, if 20% of Madison, Wisconsin residents Rode bikes for trips under 5 miles each year, carbon dioxide emissions would be reduced by more than 57,000 tons.

A 2017 research in Stockholm also indicated that the county might save 449 years of life each year if drivers who lived within a half-hour bike ride of their place of employment commuted by bike rather than by automobile. But, again, this is because fewer emissions would be produced.

These projections are not just hypothetical's. For example, the bike-sharing program in Barcelona lowers carbon dioxide emissions by around 10,000 tons annually.

What is the simplest method to start?

Your approach toward a better way of life will start with small adjustments that you are confident you can make. Consider creating "SMART" goals. SMART stands for:

- » Specific
- » Measurable
- » Attainable
- » Relevant
- » Time-bound (met by a deadline and done in a certain amount of time)

You might experience greater success if you concentrate on SMART goals. In addition, you'll be inspired to set new, more ambitious goals after your first "victory."

To start enhancing your general health, take into account the following advice.

1. Increase vegetable intake:

A study from 2010

According to a prospective study, eating more fruit and vegetables is associated with a lower risk of heart disease, stroke, cancer, and early mortality.

You don't need to eat nine servings of vegetables daily, even if eating more vegetables is better. For example, maybe you want to eat one dish of vegetables for dinner. Consider including one fruit or vegetable at each meal if you don't already.

Remember that vegetables with minimal processing are preferable. Instead of fries, try making herb-seasoned roasted potatoes or stir-frying a variety of bright veggies with a wonderful vinaigrette.

2. Introduce whole grains:

Your health will benefit if you switch to whole grains from refined ones. For example, 81 men and postmenopausal women were divided into two groups in a small 2017 study. Half of the participants consumed whole grains, while the other half consumed refined grains on a calorically equivalent diet. As a result, the whole grain group's resting metabolic rate increased after six weeks (RMR). During rest, your body expends calories or RMR.

Whole grain consumption is associated with a lower risk of diabetes, coronary heart disease, cardiovascular illness, and cancer, according to studies from 2016 and 2020.

Start by substituting one refined grain daily with whole grain; this might be your toast for breakfast or the pilaf you prepare for dinner. Then, try out various grains and flavors to see the ones you like most.

Whole grains consist of:

Plain whole grain bread, pasta, and oats

Wild and brown rice

Quinoa, farro, buckwheat, bulgur, wheat, millet, and barley

Refined grains consist of:

White spaghetti and bread

Most breakfast cereals, crisps, and white rice

pretzel\ Scrackers

3. Exercise more:

If "exercise" or "workout" makes you uncomfortable, consider this stage just moving your body.

You may stroll, ride a bike, learn how to salsa dance, practice martial arts, or sign up for an online exercise program. However, the most crucial step is to select an enjoyable pastime. The likelihood that you'll persist with an activity increases if you choose one you enjoy.

Second, remember that you don't have to start with a rigorous exercise schedule. Try to exercise for 10 minutes, five days a week. Then, add another five or ten minutes when you're ready. Continue doing this until you exercise daily for at least 30 minutes, mostly every day of the week.

4. Keep friendships:

Maintaining close friendships and regular communication with family and friends can help mental wellness.

One reason is that those who have poor connections are more likely to experience depression. For example, compared to those with the best connections, The likelihood of depression is more than twice of those in the worst relationships.

Similar to the previous point, evidence indicates that loneliness raises the likelihood of both depression and poor self-rated health. Additionally, it is linked to several health issues, including headaches, heart palpitations, and lower back, neck, or shoulder pain.

Even if you cannot meet in person, plan a weekly phone or video call to keep up with friends and family. Alternatively, just talk to a neighbor you pass by.

5. Manage your stress:

When under chronic stress, your body is always in a fight-or-flight mode. Your immune system is weakened, making you more susceptible to illnesses, such as:

Diabetes, heart disease, and intestinal issues

Depression

High blood pressure, difficulties anxiety sleeping

Through the release of stored energy, exercise can assist in alleviating stress. For example, endorphins are mood-enhancing chemicals that can be released more readily after physical activity.

Others may find relief from stress through mindfulness exercises like meditation, deep breathing, journaling, or time spent in nature. A friend's advice is also helpful.

Consider counseling if you'd like further assistance in managing your stress. You can acquire new stress-management techniques and work through issues in life by consulting with a qualified psychologist, psychiatrist, or therapist.

Exist any negative aspects?

Since everyone gets to determine what "healthy" looks and feels like for themselves, there aren't any drawbacks to living a healthy lifestyle.

This implies that you are not required to do anything that makes you unhappy. However, since we just discussed, being unhappy might impact your health.

For instance, if you dislike traditional exercise, consider other ways to move your body that you appreciate. You are not required to consume kale if you detest it.

Do I have to stop my favorite "bad behavior" now?

Living a healthy lifestyle does not require giving up activities you may view as "bad habits." For example, you can live a healthy lifestyle while enjoying cookies, skipping a workout, or drinking wine with dinner.

Occasionally indulging in pleasure can make it easier to maintain a balanced diet. However, it typically backfires to have an all-or-nothing mentality where you can only consume "good" meals and never eat "poor" ones. Being healthy includes having the freedom to savor every bite of your mother's extra-cheesy lasagna.

Days of rest are crucial for both physical and mental wellness. Excessive exercise might raise your risk of injury or lead to burnout and complete inactivity.

In addition, moderate drinking—one standard drink for women and two for men—has been related to several positive health effects. An "average drink" is:

>> 12 ounces of beer, liquid

» 5 ounces of wine

» 8 to 9 ounces of malt liquor

» Spirit, 1.5 fl oz.

Conversely, consult a medical professional if you believe you cannot stop a habit that could be harmful to your health (such as excessive alcohol use, drug use for pleasure, or smoking). They could aid in locating support.

The conclusion

A healthy lifestyle can improve your mood and lengthen your life, reduce your risk of developing certain diseases, conserve energy, and reduce your financial outlay.

Whatever you describe as a healthy lifestyle is your version of it. To be healthy, you don't need to do anything special. Instead, find out what makes you happy and gives you the most satisfaction. Then, when you make modifications, start small. Your odds of success will rise as a result, and small gains will snowball into bigger benefits.

CHAPTER 6

HUMAN HEALTH AND WAY OF LIFE

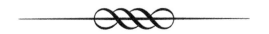

I n western civilizations, life expectancy at birth has been rising for the past century, thanks to ongoing improvements in medical care, the environment (particularly clean, safe water and food), and nutrients. For example, the life expectancy in Italy increased from 29 years in 1861 to 82 years in 2011. The exceptional longevity has also increased throughout the years. In fact, there were 165 centenarians in Italy in 1951, but there were more than 15000 by 2011. These findings were first made possible by a sharp decline in infectious illnesses, leading to sharp declines in both baby and adult mortality. In actuality, less than 10% of deaths in 2011 involved individuals under 60, compared to 74% in 1872, 56% in 1901, and 25% in 1951. However, the development in medical care for age-related illnesses, particularly cardiovascular disease and cancer, over the past few decades has allowed for a consistent extension of the longevity of 5 years over the past two decades and 2 years over the past 10 years.

These findings unequivocally demonstrate that environmental influences significantly influence human longevity and lifespan. But the increase in a lifetime in recent decades has not been followed by an equivalent increase in a healthy lifespan. In fact, the chronic nature of age- related disorders is to blame for this lifespan extension in most cases. As a result, biogerontology is currently studying interventions to increase not only a lifetime but also a healthy lifespan, or, using a new term, "health span." These therapies may be modified based on the knowledge gained from research on the genetic and biomolecular basis of longevity. In actuality, model organisms with mutations that increase lifespan lead healthy lives into old age. This implied that the genes identified as being important for life extension in both model organisms and humans may be targeted for stimulation or silencing. based on this theory, it has been reported that several genes correlated with life extension, including those related to DNA repair, stress response, immune response, and others, exhibit very different expression patterns in old age in restricted dietary mice, which live much longer and exhibit a very delayed aging phenotype than mice fed at libitum. Therefore, food restriction can cause a molecular- genetic reaction that delays aging and age-related traits. This prompted researchers to look for medications or other treatments that could affect these systems without having the negative effects of calorie restriction. We might mention protein restriction and the usage of medications targeting certain genes of the IGF-1 axis or of the FOXO/TOR pathway as some of the most significant therapies that have been considered in this context. These investigations have also made it possible to reevaluate earlier findings of regions with exceptional lifespans

Life expectancy

According to the year of birth, present age, and other demographic parameters like sex, an organism's life expectancy can be calculated statistically as the length of time on average that it is predicted to live. Life expectancy at birth (LEB), which has two definitions, is the most frequently used metric. Cohort LEB is the average lifespan of a birth cohort (all people born in a given year), and it can only be calculated for cohorts whose members have all passed away. Period LEB is the average number of years that a hypothetical cohort would live if they were subjected to the observed mortality rates from the time of their birth until their death.

Estimates of period LEB are used to calculate national LEB values for human populations supplied by national agencies and international organizations. Human LEB in the Bronze and Iron Ages was 26 years; in 2010, the world's LEB was 67.2 years. In recent years, LEB in Japan is 83, whereas it is 49 in Eswatini (Swaziland). Low LEB is caused by a combination of high infant mortality and young adult deaths caused by accidents, epidemics, plagues, wars, and childbirth before the widespread availability of modern medicine. For instance, in a society with a LEB of 40, there would be very few deaths at age 40; most deaths would occur before age 30 or after age 55.

LEB is quite sensitive to the rate of newborn mortality in populations with high infant mortality rates. This sensitivity makes LEB extremely prone to misinterpretation, causing one to believe that a population with a low LEB would have a tiny percentage of seniors. Another metric, such as life expectancy at age 5 (e5), can take infant mortality out of the equation and offer a straightforward indicator of general death rates outside of early childhood. When evaluating population structure and dynamics, aggregate population metrics like the population percentage in each age group are utilized in addition to individual-based indicators like formal life expectancy. Although this instance was uncommon, pre-modern societies generally had higher mortality rates and shorter life expectancies for both sexes at every age. A 40-year remaining period at age five may not have been unusual in communities with 30-year life expectancies, but a 60-year time span was.

Infant mortality comprised 40 and 60 percent of all deaths until the middle of the 20th century. The average lifespan between the 12th and 19th centuries, excluding child mortality, was roughly 55 years. A medieval person had a roughly 50% chance of surviving for 50–55 years, as opposed to just 25–40 years, if they made it through childhood.

According to mathematics, life expectancy is the average number of years left at a specific age. It is represented by display style e xe x,[a], which is the mean number of additional years of life for a person with certain mortality at age display style xx. Maximum lifespan, longevity, and life expectancy are not interchangeable terms. The relatively long lifespan of some people in a population is referred to as longevity. The age at death for a species' longest-living member is its maximum lifespan. An individual may pass away many years before or many years after the "anticipated" survival because the life expectancy is average.

Additionally, life tables and plant or animal ecology use life expectancy data (also known as actuarial tables). Although the related term shelf life is frequently used for consumer goods and the phrase " the concept of life expectancy may also be utilized in the context of manufactured objects.

Evolution and aging rate

Humans are among the many plants and animals with various life spans. According to evolutionary theory, organisms with genes that code for delayed aging, which frequently translates to effective cellular repair, are likely to live for a long time and escape accidents, disease, predation, etc. According to one argument, there will be less natural selection to lengthen the intrinsic life span if predation or unavoidable deaths prevent most people from living to a ripe old age. That conclusion was reinforced by Austad's well-known research of opossums, while Reznick's equally well-known study of guppies revealed the reverse association.

According to a well-known and widely accepted notion, calorie restriction—a tight budget for food energy—can increase lifespan. Many animals, most notably mice and rats, have undergone calorie restriction, which results in a nearly doubling of life span from a very low calorific consumption. Numerous recent research that relates a lower basal metabolic rate to longer life expectancy has strengthened the case for the notion. That is the secret to the long lifespan of creatures like gigantic tortoises. Studies on people who have lived at least 100 years have revealed a connection between decreasing thyroid function and their lower metabolic rate. According to an established belief, calorie restriction—a tight budget for food energy—can increase lifespan. Many animals, most notably mice and rats, have undergone calorie restriction, which results in a nearly doubling of life span from a very low calorific consumption. Numerous recent research that relates a lower basal metabolic rate to longer life expectancy has strengthened the case for the notion. That is the secret to the long lifespan of creatures like gigantic tortoises. Studies on people who have lived at least 100 years have linked their reduced metabolic rates to their decreased thyroid function.

A thorough analysis of zoo animals revealed no connection between an animal's investment in reproduction and its lifespan.

How and Why Do Life Expectancy and Aging Change?

Questions like "Why do we age?" and "How long will we live?" have been addressed in various ways since the beginning of time. Despite this legacy of interest, there hasn't been much consensus over the most important solutions to these problems. This lack of clarity has motivated many scientists to work harder, and in the last ten years or so, Regarding aging and life expectancy, there has been a tremendous increase in recent claims and studies. Unfortunately, past efforts pale in comparison, practically being obscured by these.

What sense can be drawn from this flood of fresh data? To organize the conceptual landscape and provide a context for comprehending what we have learned and have not learned, I give an overview of recent assertions regarding aging and life span in this chapter. My main goal is to support innovative research trajectories.

Recent definitions of aging include "the progressive loss of function accompanied by decreased fertility and increased mortality with advancing age." This concept, which emphasizes ever-increasing debility and ever-declining reproduction and survival rates, is contentious, especially in light of recent data on the oldest age classes in humans and several other species, which suggest that survival rates may stop declining at late ages. However, the definition of which includes a description of organismic decline, effectively captures the heart of much of the biology that sparks curiosity and drives efforts to offer a scientific explanation.

Naively, a Darwinian worldview makes aging difficult to understand.

After all, if evolution aims to produce the greatest, why might harmful traits emerge during the lifetime of an organism? Biologists have addressed the seeming Darwinian dilemma in various ways.

One of the theories offered is the "pace of living theory," which claims that animals with faster metabolic rates have shorter life spans. This claim's overall positive association is supported by

As determined by body size as a proxy, there is a correlation between metabolic rate and average life span for many creatures, particularly vertebrates. However, groupings of vertebrates show significant enough variability to call into question this theory as the only one explaining aging and life duration variations. For instance, it does not clarify why many bird species have far higher metabolic rates and longer life spans than mammals of comparable size. Nevertheless, the generally positive correlation between metabolic rate and life expectancy is strong enough to imply that metabolic variations contribute to the observed life expectancy variations among significant taxonomic groups.

The concentration of chemical byproducts damaging to the body's somatic cells increases with a greater metabolic rate, which is one possible reason explaining the link between metabolic rate and life expectancy. For instance, enzymes, particularly in the mitochondria, produce free radicals and other highly reactive molecules like hydrogen peroxide; these compounds can harm DNA and proteins. There is plenty of literature about this subject.

The "mutation accumulation theory" is another solution to the Darwinian riddle of aging, claiming that natural selection cannot prevent the accumulation of mutations with late-onset harmful consequences. This assertion is supported by the observation that later age groups are typically so tiny due to age-unrelated random mortality that natural selection's ability to eradicate harmful mutations is significantly diminished. In reality, natural selection cannot discern between the signal of harmful mutations and the signal of advantageous mutations as an organism age. According to this theory, the ability of natural selection to change phenotypes is constrained.

There is no such restriction posited in a third suggested answer to the evolutionary enigma. Instead, the "antagonistic pleiotropy theory" proposes the existence of pleiotropic mutations (those with multiple effects), which can, for example, boost early-life fertility and decrease later-life survival or fertility.

This theory proposes that aging expresses the later harmful impacts of pleiotropic mutations. Williams was the first to thoroughly develop this concept. All other variables being equal, a mutation's positive effect may outweigh its later negative effect.

The explanation is essentially the principle of compound interest, which makes it more advantageous to deposit money in the bank today rather than tomorrow. Evolution is nearly always advantageous to increasing one's children's contribution to the population earlier rather than later. For the antagonistic pleiotropy theory, there is a limitation on mutation and selection since mutations' positive and negative effects are considered inseparable, as opposed to a limitation on selection.

The "disposable soma" hypothesis further developed Williams' concept, clarifying the potential physiological mechanisms causing antagonistic pleiotropy.

They contend that as an organism age, it is favorable to conserve energy by lessening "proofreading" in somatic cells. The positive effect is that reproduction is improved because more energy is directed toward it; the adverse effect is that the soma degrades due to insufficient meticulous biochemical upkeep.

Kirkwood and Holliday's mechanistic claim is compatible with the deductions and observations that cells require proofreading because proteins and DNA are constantly being "challenged" due to the existence of free radicals in cells (see above). They go even farther, asserting that the pattern of aging we see in most animals is the outcome of an ideal equilibrium between the energy used for bodily maintenance and the energy used for reproduction. This is a powerful assertion since it indicates that the pattern of aging in a particular species results from a flawless equilibrium between somatic upkeep and reproduction. Given the fundamental limits on the creature imposed by "fixed" elements of the species like body size, mating biology, and feeding habits—aspects that serve as the backdrop for evolutionary change—such a balance cannot be improved by natural selection. Although there is evidence to back up the idea that antagonistic pleiotropy at least partially contributes to aging, there is no proof that aging is connected to an ideal balance of energy. The disposable soma hypothesis is not supported in this regard. Still, the evidence for antagonistic pleiotropy would be consistent with a weaker version of the disposable soma hypothesis, in which natural selection acts as the primary regulator of an organism's energy balance. An assertion regarding the function of natural selection differs from an assertion about optimality.

The hypotheses I've mentioned are now the most well-known, however, others have been proposed as evolutionary explanations for aging.

What is reality? Do experimental results support the mutation accumulation theory's prediction that older age groups are affected by an accumulation of mutations? Does experimental data support the antagonistic pleiotropy theory's prediction that early-life positive impacts on reproduction and survival are followed by later-life negative effects? Model organisms, particularly the nematode worm Caenorhabditis elegans, the med fly Ceratitis capitata, the fruit fly Drosophila melanogaster, and the mouse Mus musculus, have been used in the majority of contemporary experimental investigations on aging and life duration.

As a model system, each of these species has strengths and weaknesses. Therefore, most experiments concentrate mainly on either genetics or demography.

The former type of experiment today frequently entails intensive manipulation of large cohorts of people to precisely define variations in mortality and fertility rates according to age and sex. Most genetic investigations have either looked at how new mutations affect the organism's life history or how genetically altering one aspect of the life history affects another portion. To find out whether this selection produces longer-lived flies with restricted reproduction early in life, an investigator can conduct an experiment in which only longer-lived flies are permitted to produce offspring for the following generation.

The driving force is the antagonistic pleiotropy theory's prediction that mutations that increase lifespan also inescapably diminish early reproduction since more energy must be expended on surviving than reproducing (and vice versa). Alternatively, If the idea of mutation accumulation is true, selection for mutations that increase lifespan would not reduce early reproduction since these mutations would not typically have such a pleiotropic effect.

The results of certain experiments support the mutation accumulation concept. While such negative connections can be modified by evolution, it suggests that they are not the product of inescapable energy tradeoffs. Other tests confirm the antagonistic pleiotropy concept that extending life span diminishes early fertility.

Since several tests show at least some evidence of a negative correlation between survival and fertility rates, the antagonistic pleiotropy theory has greater support overall. However, this relationship is not consistently noted. Furthermore, although there is a poor correlation between fertility and survival, mutation accumulation can accelerate aging.

The latter idea has not been directly tested; thus, it is not yet obvious whether it is generally applicable.

For many investigators, Evolutionary change in life histories must be accompanied by a negative association between, for instance, early reproduction and late reproduction or survival. Otherwise, the reasoning goes, all individuals would reproduce indefinitely; Or, to put it another way, these researchers think there must be a "cost of reproduction." This mindset has the consequence that tradeoffs are "there to be found" and that the absence of evidence for them is only due to insufficient experimental power. While this reasoning is unquestionably sound in some situations, it is unclear whether it can or ought to be used as the guiding concept for all aspects of life-history development. The causes are clear-cut. If the data are interpreted literally, the causes are clear. If one accepts the data as it is and ignores preconceived notions of what "must be," one must take seriously the conflicting factual evidence on the existence of tradeoffs. Additionally, it is possible to create evolutionary models of life-history phenomena like aging and life duration in which tradeoffs do not influence key dynamics.

To properly comprehend the significance of the current body of theoretical and experimental work on aging and life duration and its limitations, it is crucial to grasp what it does and does not include. Therefore, I start by talking about the theoretical work.

Study on aging and life expectancy

As a result, non - adaptive forces such as genetic drift (evolutionary change brought on by the finite size of populations, which results in a random sampling of gametes and individuals and phylogenetic inertia (the presence of traits that have evolved in an ancestral environment or species; see Wright, 1931) are given little to no consideration in current theoretical work.

It is sometimes stated openly that evolutionary mechanisms operating at the level of the population or species could not play a significant impact, if any, in aging and life span patterns, which are thought to be the outcome of natural selection only within populations.

Second, the underlying demographic analysis of all these theories is deterministic in that it does not explicitly consider the temporal fluctuation in vital rates throughout an individual's lifespan. A major impact on the evolution of life histories and population dynamics might result from changes in, for example, the infant survival rate from one-time unit to the next or from one census to the next. These changes must be separated from longer-term variations in vital rates brought on by the waxing and waning of various lifestyles as evolution advances. The presumption that the environment is deterministic in the manner indicated above is not necessarily problematic in and of itself; many evolutionary investigations may begin with this assumption. However, assertions identifying evolutionary responses to environmental variation even though the underlying analysis does not formally account for such variation are potentially highly problematic. For instance, "Many organisms spend much of their time in highly changeable surroundings. In such conditions, we can anticipate that the co-adapted set of qualities controlling fertility and survival will have an amount of evolved plasticity that allows a variety of optimal responses appropriate for various situations." Although this assertion regarding evolution in a changeable environment is vague enough to be believable, it lacks an explicit theoretical foundation. It shouldn't be taken seriously unless supported by analyses that consider stochasticity. Why would it be a problem if these analyses were left out? Except for specific reasons revealed by a stochastic analysis, For examples of agreement and disagreement, there is no reason in general why a stochastic model's "average" behavior should even come close to matching the "average" behavior of the corresponding deterministic model. Third, aging and life expectancy are implied to evolve independently in current ideas. So, for instance, under the assumption of an arbitrarily fixed life span, the antagonistic pleiotropy theory can only reliably forecast the aging trajectory. This

51

independent evolution is conceivable in some situations, but there are other possibilities. For instance, a broader group of life-history features (such as vital rates and lifespan) may coevolved simultaneously, with none evolving before the others. It's also plausible that life span evolution is the main factor driving aging's evolution. The main message is that additional investigation of the general demographic environment for the combined evolution of aging and life expectancy is necessary. The particularity of the current explanations for how aging and life expectancy have evolved is neither exceptional relative to many other evolutionary theories nor necessarily a sign of their weakness. Because assumptions may not heavily influence forecasts, the particularity of assumptions does not always result in a particularity of predictions. But since this is not obvious, it is crucial to broaden our theoretical perspective on how aging and lifespan have changed. Such an attempt will help us better understand whether it is one in which the present theory's predictions are shown to be accurate or one in which the theory is proven to be merely a component of a more comprehensive scientific explanation of aging and the evolution of life spans.

Several issues that draw attention to significant facets of the relevant biology can be the best inspiration for developing new ideas for the evolution of aging and life span.

What is the unbiased theory of aging and lifespan to start? Such a hypothesis would forecast aging and life expectancy without using a deciding factor like natural selection. Instead, nonselective forces like genetic drift would be blamed for the patterns of aging and life span evolution. The study of molecular evolution is one area of evolutionary biology where the development of this form of neutral theory has been particularly significant.

The key justification is that competing hypotheses enhance analysis since selecting between options frequently necessitates more detailed information. Furthermore, when causal and non - causal hypotheses conflict in evolutionary biology, the value of having numerous hypotheses is further highlighted. However, as previously said, the current explanation for the evolution of aging and life expectancy almost entirely relies on natural selection acting within populations to bring about evolutionary change. One justification is the idea that vital rates, which have to do with fluctuations in population sizes, are the very things that determine evolutionary success. Accordingly, natural selection must constantly control the evolution of life's history. However, the same argument may be made regarding other life-history variables that are sometimes considered selection neutral, including the ratio of sons to daughters produced by families. Therefore, it is crucial to comprehend how aging and life expectancy can evolve without the influence of natural selection. I provide a few instances of this kind of progression below.

What is aging and life span stochastic theory? Asks the second inquiry. As was already mentioned, it can be erroneous to apply deterministic models to explain evolutionary dynamics in complex contexts. So how would a stochastic theory of aging and lifespan be "honest"? Does it open up fresh perspectives on aging and the growth of the life span?

Changes in the conclusions drawn from the deterministic theory?

Do population dynamics impact the development of aging and life expectancy? This is the third query. The phrase "population dynamics" in this context refers to long-term variations in population size. Most current theories on aging and life expectancy are based on the widespread population-genetic supposition that changes in allele and genotype frequencies alone are sufficient to characterize evolutionary change. There is no need to know the underlying demographic figures. However, depending on the accompanying aging patterns and life spans, changes in population size brought on by evolutionary change within populations may have varied effects on life histories. Therefore, a theory of aging and life span evolution that explicitly considers population dynamics is needed.

empirical studies on life duration and aging

Both our theoretical understanding of aging and the evolution of life spans and our empirical understanding of these topics still have important issues that need to be clarified.

As was already said, there has been a significant advancement in our understanding of the molecular, cellular, and genetic factors that influence aging during the past ten to fifteen years. Less focus has been placed on the factors that affect life expectancy as a whole; these factors need not be the same as those that affect aging. However, it is impressive that we now have more knowledge regarding aging. Uncertainty exists on whether our knowledge of mechanisms will truly result in a better understanding of slowing down the aging process, particularly in humans.

However, a significant improvement in our knowledge of the biology of aging and life duration at the highest biological levels has not been shown over the past ten years. Even though life expectancy and aging comparisons have been made for at least a few decades, we still lack complete data on how these characteristics are distributed. We are aware of more general patterns, such as those birds often live significantly longer than mammals of comparable size. Despite this, we know very little about the phylogenetic patterns that are aging and life span display.

The little we know in this area offers conflicting support for the current evolutionary theories of aging.

There are still many significant unanswered concerns regarding broad facets of aging and life span evolution. For instance, it is unclear whether older species tend to age more quickly.

Current theory predicts that such a correlation will occur, all other things being equal,, because an older species have had more time for natural selection to "age" it's vital rates. The use of molecular methods, which may be used to infer the relative ages of related species, is appropriate in this case. In general, it is unclear if there is a correlation between the pace of aging and the origination and extinction of species. I have given a theoretical explanation of how life span can affect the extinction rate; nevertheless, data are required to confirm or deny this relationship. Finally, and perhaps most crucially, we need to comprehend what our understanding of evolution has to say about human aging and life expectancy. There are several issues in this circumstance that need to be clarified.

Whether this distinction alters our understanding of disease dynamics and consequently affects the design of treatment programs stems from the studies of the distinction between the evolutionary dynamics of aging and those of life span described here.

Epigenome-Wide Association Studies: based on the pioneering findings that epigenetic modifications affect both the quantity (successful aging) and the course of aging, identified hundreds of sites throughout the entire genome where methylation levels differ between the oldest old and younger subjects. For example, Horwat and colleagues developed a mathematical model known as the "epigenetic clock" that demonstrated several significant aspects based on the methylation levels of 353 CpG units. First, it estimated a subject's age chronologically based on the degree of methylation in a number of his body's cells and tissues. Second, it functions as one of the most reliable age biomarkers (superior to the estimates obtained from the telomere length). Third, it was demonstrated that people with Down syndrome age more quickly, utilizing their blood and brain tissue methylation levels. Fourth, even after accounting for conventional risk factors, it could still forecast all-cause mortality.

Finally, it has been shown that the brain and muscle represent the youngest tissues of these extraordinary individuals when estimating the biological age of numerous tissues from supercentenarians.

Even though the cause-and-effect relationship between the methylation process and aging is still unclear, there is a wide range of potential applications for this discovery, from forensic uses to detailed monitoring of changes that occur with aging in specific systems or organs (muscle, brain, etc.). Future developments in this area may contribute to our understanding of the intricate physiology of aging, lifespan, and age-related illnesses for these and other reasons.

Overall, even if common variability only makes up 25% of the variation in the human lifespan, understanding the genetic factors that influence longevity may provide important clues about how to modify lifestyle to increase longevity and lengthen a healthy lifespan. A select few individuals can live a long time due to a fortunate combination of polymorphisms that enable them to have an efficient metabolism or an effective response to various stresses. By focusing on the same pathways with the proper lifestyle or therapies, most of the others can get a comparable result. In this setting, the significance of epigenetic variables will undoubtedly increase in the years to come, both as targets of therapies and as biomarkers of aging.

DNA and Human Longevity in the context of an eco-evolutionary nature-culture framework

Disentangling the causes of human lifespan, a complicated feature, will have significant theoretical and clinical implications for biomedicine. Despite several studies using various methodologies and techniques, the genetics of human lifespan is still poorly understood. Here, we contend that the extraordinarily complicated human lifespan phenotype is to blame for such a relatively underwhelming harvest. An unusual confluence of gene-environment interactions appears to cause the capacity to live into the extreme decades of the human lifespan. In light of this, a new integrative, ecological, and evolutionary perspective is offered here that describes the genetics of human longevity as a highly context-dependent phenomenon and a dynamic process, both historically and personally. Within this framework, the literature has been examined, focusing on several elements that have received relatively little consideration, including sex, individual biography, family, population ancestry, social structure, economic status, and education. Apolipoprotein E, Forkhead box O3, interleukin 6, insulin-like growth factor-1, chromosome 9p21, 5q33.3, somatic mutations, and other prominently emerged genes and regions have been highlighted, along with the strengths and limitations of the most potent and widely used tools, such as whole-genome sequencing and genome-wide association studies.

The key findings of this strategy indicate that:

1. the genetics of longevity is highly population-specific

2. small-effect alleles, pleiotropy, and complex allele timing probably play a major role

3. genetic risk factors are age-specific and need to be integrated with the context of thegeroscience perspective

4. there is a similitude between the genetics of longevity and

age-related diseases (especially cardiovascular diseases). The urgency for a worldwide approach to the mostly unstudied relationships between the three genetic components of the human body—nuclear, mitochondrial, and microbiome—is stressed in the final paragraph. We predict that the all-encompassing strategy here will contribute to an increase in the harvest above.

It is understood that long-lived mammalian species, such as naked mole rats, blind mole rats, and elephants, have acquired special features closely tied to their particular environmental niche.

Numerous researches have been conducted using animal models. Still, in this review, we will solely focus on the genetics of human longevity because, in humans, the potential to reach the extreme decades of lifespan appears to be the result of an unusual combination of gene-environment (G-E) interactions. Being a long-lived mammal, Homo sapiens most likely

Developed unusual longevity mechanisms. Because of their biological and cultural capacities for adapting to all facets of the planet and altering their settings, modern humans are characterized by a higher level of complexity. They have developed an astonishing range of adaptive cultural methods. This particular trait had and continues to significantly influence the cellular and molecular processes underlying aging and longevity. In light of this, a new integrative, ecological, and evolutionary paradigm is provided here that views the genetics of human longevity as a highly context-dependent, historically and personally dynamic phenomenon. As a result of the ongoing remodeling process, the body instituted to adjust to the degenerative changes occurring over time, which, on the other hand, happen concurrently with the changes in the environment. As a result, new GE interactions form during the lifespan. To understand the role of genetics in achieving healthy aging and extreme longevity in this complex scenario, several factors (population genetics, demography, sex, family, immunobiography, physical/geographical and cultural/anthropological environment, social networks, socioeconomic status, and education) need to be carefully considered and integrated. The genetic data were analyzed using high throughput technologies, which highlighted the relationship between population-specific dynamics and the genetics of longevity as well as the significance of small effect alleles, pleiotropy, and complex allele timing, supporting the idea that the genetic factors involved in human longevity need to be defined under a wide range of biological and non-biological variables.

Additionally, consistent with the emerging geroscience perspective, the genetics of longevity is connected to many age-related illnesses, including cardiovascular diseases (CVD). 3 According to geroscience, which has identified 7 common pillars, the mechanisms underlying aging are heavily engaged in the pathogenesis of age-related non-communicable chronic diseases (adaptation to stress, epigenetics, inflammation, macromolecular damage, metabolism, proteostasis, and stem cells and regeneration). Geroscience emphasizes that aging is the main risk factor for diseases and that diseases and their treatments speed up the aging process.4 It also provides a conceptual framework for understanding the role of genetic (protective) factors that enable a small number of people to live to the very end of their human lifespan. The plastic and intricate relationships between autosomal DNA, mitochondrial DNA (mtDNA), and microbiomes are also highlighted in this review. These relationships and somatic mutations that occur throughout a person's lifetime continuously create new and distinctive relationships between these genomes in every individual.

CHAPTER 7

HUMAN LONGEVITY'S COMPLEXITY

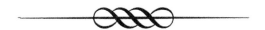

The meaning of longevity

The definition of longevity is hotly contested, and the lack of a generally accepted definition raises the risk of misunderstandings and biases when contrasting various research intended to determine the genetic influence on this attribute. Furthermore, the words lifespan, oldest old, aging, and longevity are frequently used synonymously in literature. For example, longevity is the outcome of total age class mortality selection, where cumulative mortality is historically and contextually dependent. Thus, rather than the chronological age itself, the birth cohort and the percentile of survival are two characteristics essential for the concept of longevity.

According to demographic research, there are disparities among birth cohort members who live to reach 90, 100, 105, or 110 years old, suggesting that these variances may result from significant genetic variance. 5 According to research, siblings have a higher chance of surviving into older ages as they age, indicating that hereditary factors play a greater role in survival as people age.

This finding raises the crucial point that patients who are centenarians as opposed to nonagenarians from the same birth cohort have a stronger ability to detect genetic associations with longevity. Accordingly, a recent article suggests that longevity be defined in terms of percentile survival based on the reference birth cohort for each population to avoid problems of definitional inconsistency. This suggests that the environmental context plays a crucial role in this particular phenotype. The suggested criterion to increase the likelihood of identifying genetic links is one percentile survival. The GEHA (Genetics of Healthy Ageing) Research includes nonagenarian sibling pairs to choose families enriched for genetic influences on longevity. Furthermore, familial longevity is also a criterion employed in the study of the genetics of human longevity.

Heritability and Missing Longevity Heritability

The notion of longevity opens up new discussion regarding the estimation of heredity, typically thought to be between 25% and 5% based on twin studies that only contain a small (or no) number of 90+ couples. In fact, rather than the variation of the characteristic (longevity) explained by genetic determinants, these studies likely reflect the heritability of age at death in contemporary culture.

Another study, where the authors estimated the heredity of longevity to be 16 percent, serves as an illustration of the issues and prejudice inherent in the definition of longevity in humans. The findings pointed to a strong additive genetic component, a minimal dominance effect, and no discernible epistasis in lifespan heritability. The study's digital approach to genealogical data and large sample size (3 million from an online data set of genealogy profiles of the global population) make it intriguing. Heritability calculation is based on birth cohorts from a wide range of populations between 1600 and 1910. However, no long-lived people are included (those over 100 years old were filtered out). 9 These contradictory findings introduce the growing idea of missing heritability, which is relevant to studying complicated traits like longevity. Only a small percentage of the anticipated heritability of longevity has been discovered by genomics to date. According to a recent study, the missing heritability is solely attributable to the techniques employed in the heritability computation process. In particular, the assessment of heritability relies solely on an additive model for complex traits, which disregards alternative types of inheritance patterns like epistasis. There are examples of epistatic interactions in the literature that deal with longevity. An analysis of centenarians found a substantial correlation between lifespan and the interaction of the REN gene allele and mitochondrial haplotype H, but not between the two genes examined separately.

Furthermore, unexplained environmental factors, whose connection to the genetics of human longevity will be thoroughly discussed, may distort heredity. The average differences between genotypes or the fact that each genotype displays phenotypic variance due to environmental variation cause variation between phenotypes in a population. Understanding the covariance between genes and culture, another potential bias in heritability, will require a thorough examination of variations affecting behavior and mating. Because longevity is a polygenic trait, it has been assumed that larger cohorts are required to find the variations. However, this assumption has increased cohort heterogeneity and environmental confounding factors at the expense of the biology underlying the characteristic. Finally, several writers stated that since there is growing evidence linking epigenetic inheritance with lifespan in nonhuman models, it may be necessary to look for some of the missing heritability in non-DNA characteristics that may be passed down across generations. A significant amount of work is still required to gather data on the same pool of samples, even though the analysis and integration of DNA methylation data and RNA sequencing will be useful.

CHAPTER 8

EXTREME HUMAN
LONGEVITY PHENOTYPE

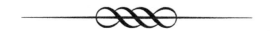

Centenarians (those over 100 years old), semi-supercentenarians (those over 105 years old), and supercentenarians (those over 110 years old) are the better research subjects for examining the genetics of human longevity because it is clear from the studies mentioned above that the genetic contribution to longevity increases with age. Characterizing the phenotype to include in the analysis is one of the new issues in genetic investigations. The word "phenomics," coined by evolutionary biologist Michael Soule, refers to all conceivable methods of describing populations and individuals. The key findings are quickly described after extensive characterization of centenarians and semi supercentenarians.

Biochemical characteristics in addition to having an excellent metabolic profile with retained glucose tolerance and insulin sensitivity and low serum levels of insulin-like growth factor (IGF)- I and IGF-II, centenarians have a phenotype comparable to that of calorie-restricted individuals.

Prevalence of age-related disorders: Centenarians significantly shorten the time they spend disabled25, and they postponed or avoided most major age-related diseases.

26–30 People who live over the age of 105 are also phenotypically considerably more similar to one another than younger people who pass away in their 80s and 90s, which is consistent with the compression of morbidity scenario.

Epigenetics: The epigenetic clock found that the DNA methylation ages of centenarians declined, showing that they are physiologically younger than their chronological age

Metabolomics: Researchers have discovered the first metabolomic signature of healthy aging by examining the plasma and urine of Italian centenarians and their descendants. In North Italian centenarians, certain sphingolipids and glycerophospholipids have been identified, along with a drop in tryptophan levels. 32 Through particular modification of the arachidonic acid metabolic cascade and increased cytochrome P450 (CYP) enzyme activity, this centenarian's metabolomic signature revealed distinctive changes in pro-and anti-inflammatory chemicals detoxification.

The biology of circadian rhythms is a newly discovered factor in familial lifespan that is probably regulated by genetic makeup and social and environmental factors. Even though the data are currently scant and sometimes pertain to a small number of people, circadian rhythms, Including central (placed in the suprachiasmatic nucleus) and peripheral clocks, degrade with age. However, they appear to be well retained in centenarians, including sleep. Compared to the general population, studies on the offspring of long-lived subjects revealed intact rhythmicity of serum non-high-density lipoprotein cholesterol content, and centenarians exhibit decent sleep quality. In humans, the genetics of circadian rhythms is quite population-specific. According to a mouse study, SIRT1 is the gene that regulates both longevity and circadian rhythms, and raising SIRT1 levels in mice with genetically altered brains appears to slow the decline of circadian functions with aging.

Controls in the Genetics of Longevity Defined

A very difficult problem in the study of the genetics of lifespan is how to define controls. It's noteworthy that the studies can be split into two primary categories:

1. Research including younger, healthy controls from the same family or the broadercommunity

2. Research involving patients with age-related illnesses, presuming that these illnesses, as recently claimed, constitute a condition of accelerated aging. The new age of molecular biomarkers of aging, which introduce the idea of biological age, is also leading to the emergence of a new definition of controls (described in the section Perspectives).

Healthy Individuals as Controls Younger Than Cases (Centenarians as a Case Study)

The selection of controls for the study of sporadic longevity was difficult and contentious. As soon as the threshold for longevity was established, numerous researchers randomly chose unrelated individuals from the general population as controls, presuming that the likelihood of centenarians in the control group was low due to the rarity of the trait. On the other hand, the power of a study can be increased by choosing a group of control subjects who did not live past the average life expectancy of their demographic cohort. By doing this, the potential enrichment of longevity variations in the control group is reduced.

According to a recent paper, both approaches offer advantages and disadvantages. Still, in both instances, the results could be skewed due to the centenarians' and controls' distinct birth cohorts.

CHAPTER 9

GERIATRICS AND GERONTOLOGY

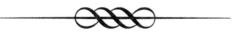

R esearch into and management of the "longevity revolution" and
"population aging."

Geriatrics: What is it?

The Greek words "Geron" (for "old man") and "Patricia" (for "art of healing") are translated as "the study of old age's medical aspects and the application of aging's biological, behavioral, and social elements to older people's care, prevention, diagnosis, and treatment."

The second part of this definition refers to the knowledge acquired in a different academic field called gerontology, which is defined as the theoretical study of old age or "the study of aging from the broadest perspective" (Greek: logos, "speech, reason, the study").

Both phrases were developed in the early 20th century, but "geriatric" understanding of specific illnesses affecting older people stretches back to Hippocrates and Galen, the two men who established Western medicine. Wards, societies, and associations were the first institutional academic foundations for geriatric medicine, although they didn't emerge until the 1930s. The same is true for gerontology, which made its debut at this time as a science with the associated institutional and academic institutions. For instance, the German Society for the Study of Aging was established in 1938 and reemerged as the German Society of Gerontology in 1966.

A core description of the "mechanistic principle" is that biological aging is the gradual buildup of molecular damage in cells and tissue while cellular healing mechanisms deteriorate. As a result, cells, tissues, and organs become less functional, making them more susceptible to illness, harm, and demise. Examples include DNA damage, improper protein synthesis, and the cross-linking of protein molecules, which can result in plaques in neurons or the hardening of arteries, among other things. Many biogerontologists think that such damaged molecules and age-related disorders are related causally.

This prompts the query of whether aging itself ought to be treated as a sickness.

The idea that aging is a disease was widely held and dominant from Roman antiquity until the early 20th century when contemporary geriatrics and gerontology brought about a change. The disciplines' founders distinguished between "normal" and "pathological" aging as a key component of their beliefs. This distinction should assist the objective of 'normal' aging support and 'pathological' aging prevention. In addition, two of the most well-known theories of health also support the distinction between disease and aging.

On the other hand, the idea that aging is a sickness based on its symptoms and the pain it causes is prevalent in bioethics. Some biogerontologists have made a similar argument, concluding that because of the causal relationship between age-related molecular alterations and age-associated disorders founded on the "mechanistic principle," aging itself should be viewed as a disease.

Biogerontologists contend that it would be crucial to treat aging as a disease for practical regulatory considerations, such as ensuring that new interventions that claim to decrease aging are examined in accordance with the regulatory standards for clinical trials. According to a recent remark, the Food and Drug Administration might be amenable to such a proposal.

In biogerontology, the opposite viewpoint that distinguishes between disease and aging appears to be in the minority nowadays.

The term "non-genetic principle" alludes to Rattan's second principle, which rejects the idea that biological aging is genetically programmed but does not completely rule out the possibility that longevity and aging may have a genetic component. In some of the older ideas of biological aging, a genetic program resembling that utilized for growth and development was assumed to exist. However, the use of the word "non-genetic" idea makes it obvious that most researchers in contemporary biogerontology disagree with this.

Genetic effects that hasten aging can exist even with no hereditary aging program. An illustration of this idea is the idea known as "antagonistic pleiotropy," which holds that some genes may have earlier beneficial effects that outweigh later negative consequences. For instance, a genetic background for an active immune system may offer short-term protection from infectious infections but long-term auto-immune reactions and inflammations. There is also proof that longer lifespan have a genetic component. According to studies, there is a higher chance that a person's close relatives will live to be very old.

An illustration of this idea is the idea known as "antagonistic pleiotropy," which holds that some genes may have earlier beneficial effects that outweigh later negative consequences. For instance, a genetic background for an active immune system may offer short-term protection from infectious infections but long-term auto-immune reactions and inflammations. There is also proof that longer lifespans have a genetic component. According to studies, there is a higher chance that a person's close relatives will live to be very old. Furthermore, after a certain amount of time, organisms of a species frequently pass away from external factors (such as malnutrition, extreme cold, or predators). For instance, after a year, 90% of mice in the wild pass away. Therefore, if certain mice with genetic modifications lived longer but generated fewer offspring, they would soon vanish from the wild. This line of reasoning also suggests that the occurrence of old age or weakness is not natural. Alternately, "the amount of maintenance is the aim for natural selection, not aging," as the biogerontologist phrased it. According to biology, a person's life is split into three phases: the "developmental span," the "adult span," which is further subdivided into a "health span," and the "senescent span," which is characterized by disorders that are linked to aging.

Last but not least, the molecular and genetic elements of biological aging point to potential targets for novel therapies based on biogerontological research. These interventions, which affect various biological aging processes to slow down or delay the changes associated with those processes, have been successfully used in laboratory organisms, including mammals like mice, rats, and monkeys, as well as more basic organisms like yeast nematodes, or fruit flies. These changes have increased the lifetime and health of those creatures.

The average human life duration will be increased, either little or significantly, if aging is slowed or stopped. The term "moderate life extension" refers to the continuation of the previous trend that characterized the first longevity revolution. For instance, the outcome might gradually increase the average life expectancy from its present level of 80 years to its current maximum of 120 years. A "radical life extension" would result if aging could be drastically slowed down, stopped, or even reversed. Any significant rise above the current maximum life span would fall within this category. It is significant to highlight that the emergence of morbidity in old age must also be considered with increased human longevity. A shorter, similar, or longer period during which persons experience age-related disorders may be connected with longer life spans.

Morbidity compression

The amount of time that would be increased and the period of life that would be impacted—such as the developmental span, health span, or senescent span—must be taken into account. The obvious objective, which corresponds to the highly praised objective of a "compression of morbidity," is to increase the health span at the expense of the senescent span.

Argues for the purposeful extension of senescence, citing this possibility as one of the risks associated with anti-aging therapies.

Biologists dispute that this is a likely consequence, claiming that it is inconsistent with the findings of animal tests and that the senescent span cannot be endlessly prolonged relative to the "health span." Combined objectives of aging interventions: a foundation for ethical analysis and evaluation

Some of these objectives and associated priorities are more debatable than others. In general, it is seen to be preferable to prevent age-related disorders from reducing morbidity. This is regarded as the main argument for intervening in biological aging because it is thought that intervention for its own sake is more troublesome. The same holds for a further increase in human life expectancy. Concerns increase as the potential for delaying aging and prolonging life becomes more extreme. Therefore, a moderate scenario that would be widely accepted is extending the health span at the expense of the senescent span without increasing the present average life span. This would be in line with the first notion of a "compression of morbidity," promoted by James F. Fries in the 1980s and elevated to a significant public policy objective in light of population aging. However, biogerontologists believe it is unlikely that a slower aging process would decrease morbidity without an increase in longevity. The average life duration will rise if health improves as people age.

The onset of senescence will either be simply delayed, or the age-related morbidities may last longer but be less severe — a condition known as a "dynamic equilibrium."

The scenario put up by advocates of the longevity dividend combines morbidity compression with a modest seven-year increase in human life expectancy. In the upcoming decades, this might be accomplished by reducing biological aging.

Aubrey de Grey also asserts that those who will experience halted and even reversed aging have already been born, which is a more contentious claim. His case is predicated on the idea that various forms of cellular and molecular damage are the root of biological aging. These are well-known, and it is already known how to fix them. The next step would be to conduct organized experiments to use these techniques.

The right distinctions between these objectives and forecasts must be made in ethical assessments of the "second longevity revolution." The concepts and practices of biogerontology, population aging, and the multidisciplinary perspectives of geriatrics and gerontology on aging and old age should also be considered. However, the bioethical debate has thus far largely concentrated on aspects of radical life span extension, such as the attainment of "immortality" through halted aging. This also holds for the few ethics advisory board papers that discuss the possibility of a "second longevity." Ethical considerations: overviews and reports on age-related therapies and life extension by expert groups

Robert Veatch, a bioethicist, compiled a collection of essays on life-extension technologies in 1979. The authors were mostly associated with the Hastings Center.

It's interesting to note that the Hastings Center's study team on "Death and dying" observed enough advancement in pertinent biotechnologies to spark several important queries about the necessity of extending human life. As a result, many of the fundamental abstract values that are pertinent in this situation are already covered in this volume.

It discusses whether it is desirable to extend human life further, whether death is bad, whether aging is an illness, and whether ensuring that everyone has access to life-extension technologies is a prerequisite of justice.

The (US) President's Council on Bioethics is the next significant organization interested in the topic of extended lifespan attained via procedures that either halt or arrest aging. The 2004 book Beyond treatment discusses advancements in human improvement, and the chapter "Ageless bodies" considers the potential effects of a "second longevity revolution." The paper distinguishes between personal and social issues. It examines both, focusing on the relevance of a "natural life span" (equivalent to the existing average life span) for a "happy life."

A book on the idea of radical life extension, the so-called "fountain of youth," edited by bioethicists Stephen G. Post and Robert N. Binstock, has also been released. It features contributions from a variety of academic disciplines. Many authors have contributed further to discussions on "radical life span extension." The National Intelligence Council finally released a report on six technologies that could upend US society in 2008. This research addresses the issue of equal access to these cutting-edge technologies and imagines more widespread economic and cultural effects if biotechnology is employed to extend human life.

One may anticipate that there would be additional studies and summaries over the next 30 years, given the significant changes that a second longevity revolution could bring about for both people and societies. However, these studies also mainly concentrate on abstract qualities and the merits of drastic life span extensions. They are less conscious of the aging population and the existing social environment. The World Health Organization, the European Commission, and the House of Lords have asked expert committees to prepare findings on problems associated with the challenges of population aging. It is essential that the work of national and international authorities and organizations be taken into account in the systematic ethical evaluation of a potential increase in longevity by slowed aging (and vice versa). The same holds for conceptions that support modest biogerontological outlooks, such as the longevity dividend program and moderate life span extensions.

The same frequently holds for certain bioethical authors who have written about the topic.

Ethical considerations: a personal viewpoint The personal benefit of longer life Would it be beneficial for people to live longer if aging happened more slowly? Before moving on to the social dimensions, such as the benefits to or burdens on societies, or justice issues, one must first evaluate the ethical implications of a potential second longevity revolution. Arguments over whether longer lifespans and slower aging are good or bad can be categorized using a popular ethical theory distinction. Utilitarian approaches allow them to be based on utility in terms of pleasure and suffering. Finally, the conditions for a rich or fulfilling human life are discussed about notions of the good life.

Finally, arguments based on obligations might be made in the context of deontological ethics. If these arguments apply to either moderate or extreme life extension, they can be further distinguished (slower or arrested aging).

Arguments for moderate life extension based on utility

As mentioned above, modest life extension would maintain the first longevity revolution's trend, resulting in a gradual rise in the average life expectancy over the following decades. If the research from biogerontology is to be believed, slowing aging will probably result in better health as people age and longer lifespans. In addition to citing the high value placed on longevity across cultures, proponents of this outlook can also point to a shorter suffering from age-related illnesses and a longer sense of joy that can be added over a longer life.

These arguments are difficult to refute based on utility. It is feasible to counter that the aggregate perspective is unfounded and that if additional years are added to the present life duration, there are no appreciable gains in relevant experience. It might also be claimed that as long as it is not certain whether compression of morbidity can be achieved, the suffering will just be delayed. However, even though these arguments seem centered on utility and easing pain, they are implicitly founded on presumptions about the "ideal life" for human longevity.

CHAPTER 10

GENETICS OF LONGEVITY: ECOLOGICAL INSIGHTS

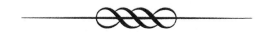

What is Ecology?

E cology is a branch of science, including human science, population, community, ecosystem and biosphere. Ecology is the study of organisms, the environment and how the organisms interact with each other and their environment. It is studied at various levels, such as organism, population, community, biosphere and ecosystem.

An ecologist's primary goal is to improve their understanding of life processes, adaptations and habitats, interactions and biodiversity of organisms

It is well known that a complex interplay between environment, genetics, and stochastic factors affects lifespan. Ecological models, which are infrequently taken into account in studying human longevity, appropriately consider such complexity. According to the evolutionary theory of niche construction, a person's genetic makeup may interact with their surroundings and the outside world. As a result, we'll consider the interaction with the environment to be the red herring in our examination of the genetics of longevity. We assume that all potential interactions may change depending on the unique traits of each individual to comprehend this complicated ecology. As a result, we begin by describing each person's biological identity, which is based on innate traits (such as sex and uncommon variations) and attributes acquired throughout a lifetime (such as somatic mutations and immunologic stimuli that constitute immunobiography). (ecological space), we present three dimensions that can accommodate the various timescales of interactions between genes, culture, and ecology: human population genetics (population genetics and population-specific G-E interactions); the genetics of families (assortative mating or indirect effects of parents' genotypes);

Socio - economic variables and lifespan genetics

Individual Variability in Longevity Genetics

» Immunobiography as an Example of Biological Biography

Immunity

Immunity can be defined as a complex biological system endowed with the capacity to recognize and tolerate whatever belongs to the self, and to recognize and reject what is foreign (non-self).

According to the ecological viewpoint, genetic and environmental factors interact dynamically to determine how long people live. Since each person's genetic makeup and particular life experiences combine to create a unique signature, G-E interactions in centenarians are particularly peculiar to each individual. This idea has been named "immunologic biography" because it was developed from an immunologic point of view. The immune system components, which include innate and adaptive, can remember all the immunologic encounters and stimuli it has been exposed to because of its memory and plasticity. Immune responses are influenced and shaped by at least two dimensions: (1) space, which is made up of relationships between people and their unique environments, according to geography and history of the population they belong to (pathogens, nutrition, climate, way of life, among other things); and

(2) time, as each person is the product of time-dependent adaptive processes (such as immunosenescence and inflammaging).

These ideas can also be applied to other bodily systems and organs, such as the brain, endocrine system, and gut microbiota, which can keep track of past lifelong stimuli and contribute to the formation of an individual's biological biography that affects aging and its trajectory from early in life.

Germline (Rare Variants) and acquired (Somatic) Mutations: Individual Genetic Identity

Each person has a distinct genetic makeup with a particular blend of common and rare or even private de novo variants (germline variations), making each person's genetic identity a dynamic process. At the same time, somatic mutation accumulation is seen as people age. These genetic variation combinations make up the unique genetic identity, which is constantly changing as we age.

It is difficult to research unusual variations in aging and longevity because these traits are inherently rare. Two basic strategies can be considered in this regard: (1) to examine the results of these variants when large-scale DNA sequencing and focused molecular investigations are combined (2) to examine population isolates. Due to the genetic homogeneity of these populations, which makes it possible for rare variants to have increased in frequency, this method has successfully identified rare variants associated with complex phenotypes. In fact, the effect of random genetic drift on increasing allele frequencies is greater for rare variants than for common variants.

Somatic mosaicism, a lifetime phenomenon in all human tissues that occurs from fertilization until death, is another factor that influences genetic identity. In addition to mistakes in the DNA duplication process, DNA double-strand breaks, ineffective DNA repair, and abnormal chromosomal segregation, this accumulation is brought on by exposure to external agents (such as ultraviolet light and pollution). According to a study on Italian centenarians, the buildup of unrepaired DNA damages, the loss in DNA repair effectiveness, and replicative senescence are well-established aspects of aging. 64 A detailed account of the relationship between somatic mutations in autosomal DNA and clonal hematopoiesis, which constitute a developing link between lifespan and CVD, is presented in Somatic Mutations and Clonal Hematopoiesis.

Numerous aging studies have shown that somatic mosaicism of mtDNA, also known as heteroplasmy, shows a buildup of mtDNA mutations in healthy individuals as they age. In addition, a study on female centenarians and their of fspring that used an ultradeep DNA sequencing approach capable of detecting low-frequency alleles revealed a heteroplasmy profile unique to each individual (private component) and the presence of heteroplasmy shared between centenarian mothers and daughters within each family.

CHAPTER 11

HUMAN LONGEVITY AND
SEXUAL DIMORPHISM GENETICS

I t is well known that, with a few notable exceptions, human longevity is strongly correlated with sex and that women typically live longer than men. This is probably due to a combination of biological and social factors, as is evidenced by the survival rate in Italy per 100,000 people of various ages. Males are denoted in blue, while females are denoted in red. The triangle on the left shows how genetics have a role in the lifespan attribute. B, The upper heatmap demonstrates that the ratio of Italian women to men who are centenarians rises from north to south (Passarino et al. 66). Italy's genetic variation on the Y chromosome is depicted in the lower map (Boattini et al. 2013292). The squares' sizes are proportional to the absolute value of the SPCA scores. Black squares reflect positive values of the spatial principal component analysis (SPCA), while white squares represent negative values. The Italian population has a clearly defined distribution of sex, cultural and socioeconomic structures, and autosomal and uniparental genetic variations.

The inheritance of remarkable longevity is also influenced by gender.

Maternal and paternal inheritances are likely to contribute to exceptional life in males, according to an examination of the parental age of an Ashkenazi Jewish cohort with exceptional longevity. However, maternal inheritance appears to be more significant in females. Studies on evolution offer hints about how to understand these sex-specific influences.

First, as evidenced by the Korean population of eunuchs, sex hormones, particularly the elimination of testosterone at young ages, have been shown to extend lifespan in mammals and humans.

The trade-off between immunological investment and features that increase competitive success in males has influenced genetic variation in the genes responsible for testosterone levels throughout human evolution. According to the resource's allocation theory, testosterone significantly contributes to muscular male growth while suppressing immunological responses (testosterone is regarded as an immunosuppressant).

Second, sex differences are influenced by cultural variables. For example, when scientists discovered that Hadza hunter-gatherers (Tanzania) moms had to choose between gathering food for themselves and caring for newborns, the grandmother hypothesis gained traction in 1980. Because healthy women may have improved the reproductive success of their offspring, caring for their grandchildren, this cultural process—observed exclusively in humans—may have molded genetic polymorphisms imparting sex-specific advantage for survival after menopause.

Third, since mtDNA is inherited from the mother, only females may directly and adaptively respond to selection through females, as experimental research on Drosophila has shown. This means that neutral or advantageous mutations for females might accumulate in the population and hurt males (a phenomenon known as the Mother Curse). This is because men are typically constrained by the number of mating. In contrast, females might have a limited number of offspring due to physiological factors (number of gametes and energetic expenditures of each pregnancy). According to a recent study that revealed an accumulation of harmful mutations in genes primarily expressed in men, this results in different selection dynamics in females than in males. According to the research of Camus et al., the mitochondrial genome is a hotspot for mutations that impact sex-specific aging patterns and result in sexual dimorphism in old age.

Additionally, a key factor in determining the variation in penetrance and expression of mitochondrial illnesses with different trends in different sexes is the interaction between nuclear DNA and the mitochondrial genome (referred to as mitonuclear interactions). The accumulation of mtDNA mutations that affect the functionality of oxidative phosphorylation exerts strong selective pressure on the nuclear genome to make compensatory changes that restore the damaged function.

The mechanics of evolution optimize fitness following reproductive efficiency. Due to physiological limitations on the number of gametes and the energy expenditure of pregnancy, females can only have a certain number of children. In contrast, men are constrained by the number of matings (down part of the figure). Because the number of reproductively active females is the limiting element determining the number of newborns for each generation, evolution heavily favored female fitness. This distinction inevitably results in sex-specific selective pressures on the mitochondrial and nuclear genomes that are stronger in females than in males. Nuclear DNA is referred to as DNA, and mitochondrial DNA is mtDNA.

Data from Drosophila melanogaster indicated that sex significantly impacts this process. According to research on isonuclear fly lines in which different mitochondrial haplotypes were inserted into a predetermined foreign nuclear background, a breakdown of the coevolved mitonuclear genotype results in sterility in males but not females.

The study of human longevity genetics has only lately begun to consider the dimorphism in longevity. In the GEHA investigation, 90+ male (N pairs=263) and female (N pairs=1145) sib pairs underwent a linkage analysis, and 3 loci that were sex-specifically associated with lifespan were found: 8p11.21-q13.1 (men), 15q12-q14 (women), and 19q13.33-q13.41 (women) (women). 8 In a population of more than 2200 Chinese centenarians, a recent genome-wide association study (GWAS) study82 looked at the connection with longevity separately in men and women. Although several intriguing sex-specific longevity variants were found, the authors could not identify any locus related to lifespan above the official 10-8 GWAS threshold. The polygenic risk score used in the study suggests that various pathways affect both men's and women's longevity. For instance, pathways related to inflammation and immunology were shown to be more prevalent in men. In contrast, pathways related to PGC-1 (PPAR coactivator-

Function and tryptophan metabolism were more prevalent in women. It is important to note that the GWAS approach probably restricted the sex-specific longevity study because of the clear fall in cohort size when split into males and females.

Genetics of Longevity and Familial Ecology

Most publications on the genetics of human longevity begin with the phrase "Longevity runs in families," and families fill a certain ecological niche. One of the early pieces of evidence comes from research using a geographical-genealogical method on the Sardinian community (Italy). These studies demonstrated two things: (1) a non-random distribution of centenarians by place of birth and peculiar area (in the province of Nuoro) of exceptional male longevity is identified and called the blue zone83; and (2) longevity clusters in families and occur among the ascendants of a specific branch of the family. 84 Children born to moms who later lived to be 100 years old had significantly lower infant mortality than children born to mothers from the same cohorts. Still, they did not live to be 100 years old, an odd feature of Sardinian familial longevity. According to a study of 1700 sibships from families of centenarians in the New England Centenarian Study, a history of familial longevity increases the chances that a person would live a long life. Furthermore, compared to age-matched controls born from parents who passed away before living to the predicted lifespan for their cohort, the offspring of centenarians exhibit improved health conditions.

However, families are shaped not only by genes but also by cultural and ecological dynamics, particularly in small populations that uphold local customs and where weddings occur within the same (or, at the very least, close) small communities (such as in Nuoro).

Two studies in various communities, including the Dutch and the Calabrian, illustrate the impact of social and family structure on the genetics of longevity (South Italy). The first study discovered that spouses of long-lived partners did not exhibit any advantage in terms of survival, despite spending most of their adult lives with their partner. This finding suggests that the effect observed was primarily due to hereditary factors. In contrast, female spouses of long- lived siblings in Southern Italy (Calabria) also live longer than those in the same birth cohort, suggesting that women may benefit more than men from a hospitable environment to reach a century of age.

These findings are the study's strength since they made it clear to what extent the study of longevity genetics may be influenced by familial, social, and anthropological behaviors. In addition, spouses of members of long-living families tend to be healthier than sex- and age- matched members of the general population, according to the Long-Life Family Research (LLFS), a longitudinal family-based study of longevity and healthy aging. 90 These observations may have a genetic component to the underlying mechanism. Assortative mating based on traits that have strong hereditary components, such as anthropometric measurements, behavior, educational attainment, and cognitive ability, maybe a process. Ancestry-related assortative mating also occurs in families chosen for longevity, as seen by the high genetic similarity of spouse pairings, especially for older generations. The first assortative mating experiments and hypotheses were made in 1914. They were founded on the idea that longevity within a family was something to be proud of. Assortative mating is phenotype-based (driven by various factors, such as educational level, socioeconomic status, language, behavior, culture, etc.) as opposed to high levels of inbreeding, which affects the frequency of each locus independently and can transform linkage disequilibrium and the genotype frequency distribution of the loci implicated in the assortment to an excess of homozygozity Accordingly, a recent study revealed that genetic variations connected to education predict longevity, indicating that people with a higher number of education-related genetic variations had parents who lived longer. The parental genomes, typically neglected in genetic studies, also appear to be important because non-transmitted alleles can influence a kid through their effects on the parents and other family members, a phenomenon known as genetic nurturing.

Population Approach to Genetics of Longevity

Numerous studies have shown that longevity is greatly influenced by the setting. A novel finding is that genes and processes that affect longevity are also population-specific. The study on longevity in the Chinese population found unusual, context-dependent pathways related to lifespan. Longevity is probably a population-specific phenomenon that involves both public and private mechanisms. It is a convergent phenotype that is achieved through context-specific (genetic and nongenetic) mechanisms that are partially public (at least for biological functions) and partially private for each population.

Within this perspective:

The fast-changing and population-specific environmental variables can have a significant impact on G-E interactions, causing the same alleles to have distinct effects in other populations;

Because of evolutionary dynamics like demographic history, migration, bottlenecks, drift, or positive selection that was performed in the past, allele frequency can attain high frequency in some populations.

The first scenario is illustrated by TCF7L2 rs7903146-TT, the most significant genetic marker of T2D Mellitus associated to cardiovascular events. According to the research of Corella et al.

1997., the Mediterranean diet can offset the risk genotype's effect on stroke risk, indicating that a genetic connection can be affected by population-specific environmental factors.

A genetic study on the Italian population illustrated the second scenario, whereby the frequency of variations linked to various diseases displayed varying patterns depending on previous environmental selective forces. The study by Sazzini et al. examined more than 500 000 SNPs in 780 individuals drawn from the Italian population and showed how, when taking into account the North to South cline, local historical adaptations and various admixture events with continental and Mediterranean populations shape the frequency of risk variants for complex pathologies like T2D Mellitus and CVD. In the investigation of the genetics of longevity, variation from within populations is not the only source to consider. There have been reports of minor but consistent changes in allele frequencies among populations that are geographically close to one another but have different ecoregions, food compositions, and modes of subsistence. As a result, certain populations in various geographic locations that share the same environment may increase the frequency of the same adaptive allele. The APOE situation is illustrative and is discussed in more detail below. The Y chromosome and mtDNA must be considered in the same ways, and mitonuclear coadaptation coevolutionary trajectories are likely to be population specific.

Different Socioeconomic Settings and the Genetics of Longevity

Another niche human has created, the social and ecological component is important in the genetics of complex features. It is well recognized that socioeconomic circumstances can have an effect on aging and human longevity. One of the most startling examples of longevity comes from Glasgow, where persistently impoverished regions have been linked to higher rates of mortality. Korea is one hundred examples. where the population's economic situation rapidly improved, making South Korea one of the most developed countries. On the other hand, NorthKorea continues to have one of the poorest populations. The population of North Korea had 0.7centenarians per million in 1925 and 2.7 centenarians per million in 2010, while the population of South Korea had 2.7 centenarians per million in 1925 and 38.2/1 million in 2010. 101 These demographic statistics provide fresh information for studying the genetics of human longevity because they show how social factors can alter the genetic influence within a population. This was shown in a study by Rumsfeld et al. 102. They examined 12 500 people from Estonia and showed that, during the Soviet era, 2% of the variation in schooling and success was due to genetic factors; however, following independence, this percentage rose to 6%. 102 Illegitimacy of the birth and parental occupation (especially paternal one), according to two recent studies that examined the influence that socioeconomic situation at birth exerts on whole life mortality, were linked to an increase in mortality at all ages. 103,104 The most straightforward explanation for these discrepancies is that socioeconomic status affects nutritional profile, stress levels, and infection exposure. However, recent data revealed that epigenetic modifications (particularly DNA methylation) may recode information of the father's environmental exposure and then be transmitted to the offspring,105-107 supporting the crucial role of evaluating these factors for the missing heritability.

Furthermore, it has been hypothesized that maintaining social ties can help people live longer108 and is linked to lower mortality, even if social contacts tend to decline as people age. In fact, a meta-analysis of 308 849 people who were observed for an average of 7.5 years showed that people with social contacts have a higher likelihood of surviving (by 50%) than people with few and poor social interactions. 109 On the other hand, a higher propensity for depression among the elderly can be linked to a lack of connections with the family, particularly with grandkids. 110 Even though a function in these social interactions may be hypothesized, data on behavioral genetics' role in determining them have not been studied. In actuality, genes may undergo positive selection based on how they influence social behavior (also called indirect effect because they confer a characteristic crucial to boosting social interactions). The language gene FOXP2, which indirectly enhances the probability of social interactions between individuals and probably increases their frequency due to the advantage in social conduct, is the most prominent example is the study of human evolution.

Similarly, under the influence of social selection, genes linked to testosterone underwent significant alteration during evolution to enable social interactions during the transition from nomadic to stable communities (more numerous). Conclusion: (1) According to the findings of the Health and Retirement Survey in the United States111, the process of remodeling and the genes favoring longevity (or predisposing to serious chronic health conditions) appear to be different in different socioeconomic backgrounds; (2) New socioeconomic conditions have recently emerged, such as the obesogenic environment. As a result, genes that encourage healthy aging today likely differ from genes that favor longevity a century ago (for example, during the First World War or when antibiotics were not invented).

The Main Results from Whole-Genome Sequencing in the Genetics of Human Longevity

Whole-genome sequencing is now the most illuminating method for genetic study. In addition, researchers now have additional options for genetic studies thanks to recent developments in sequencing technologies and the decrease in sequencing prices.

Although candidate gene analysis was used in the initial studies on the genetics of human longevity, the current methodology relies on genome-wide approaches to identify the most useful loci, with functional tests conducted both in vitro and in vivo as the final step of the analysis. Whole-genome sequencing's key benefit is that it enables the analysis of each person's particular genomic variability (both in coding and non-coding areas) without imputation, which may introduce bias due to the reference population. The few whole-genome sequencing studies on the genetics of human longevity that are now accessible are as follows: (1) the initial investigations, carried out by Sebastiani et al. and Ye et al, examined a small number of people who had reached the extreme decades of life. The Sebastiani study, published in 2011, sequenced two supercentenarians (those older than 110 years old). Still, the small sample size

Precluded statistical analysis. However, an intriguing finding was that the two patients probably represented two different approaches to surviving into old age. The female had large regions of homozygosity on several chromosomes, indicative of inbreeding among her ancestors. She only possessed five of the 16 frequent variations identified in GWAS studies as being connected with long life and metabolism. The same research in males revealed 11 of the 16 frequent variations related to longevity and no corresponding stretches of homozygosity.

» These findings indicated that the woman was enriched for unique mutations that increase longevity (because of her familial genetic background).

» Due to the uniqueness of the data, the second study (113), which took into account amonozygotic twin pair living to 100 years of age, also looked into the frequency of somatic mutations.

» Gierman et al. third's investigation, published in 2014,114, examined 17 supercentenarians (those over 110 years old)

with European ancestry. Still, the effectiveness of the analysis was diminished by the inclusion of publicly accessible genetic data as a control (reducing the number of variants to analyze). The following summary of the key findings:

1. The gene with the highest enrichment for rare protein-altering variants in this cohort of supercentenarians was TSHZ3. Still, the replication in the second cohort of 99 long-lived individuals failed.

2. There was no substantial indication of enrichment in supercentenarians for a single uncommon protein-altering variant or for genes hosting rare protein-altering variants as compared to controls.

3. Erikson et al's recent publication, which likewise had the greatest sample size, was released in 2016; however, the authors focused on a healthy aging phenotype (dubbed Wellderly by the author) in participants who were 84.29.3 years old. The study's age range suggests that little research on lifespan has been done. 116 The key finding of this study is the correlation between loci in the COL25A1 gene, which codes for a protein produced in the brain and linked to amyloid plaques, and healthy aging.

Thus, sequencing research on lifespan is developing. Still, the data that was accessible prevented a true discovery phase when compared to the data that was already available. In addition, the interpretation of the sequencing data is hampered by the small sample size and absence of controls.

Overview of Human Longevity Genetics

The right way to define phenotypes for genetic investigations

1. Demographic factors are used to define longevity (1 percentile survival)

2. Demographic factors are used to define longevity (1 percentile survival)

3. Stay away from basing your notion of lifespan on self-reported data.

4. As a paradigm of accelerated aging, controls can include healthy people, family members, and those with age-related illnesses.

5. The definition of controls needs to take biological age into account.

6. Males and females have differing lifespans

7. When the sample size is large enough, the genetic analysis must be carried out separately formales and females.

The environmental viewpoint

The genetics of longevity is not a static concept, and a protective/risk allele must be combined with other facts that describe the individual over a specific time period.

1. (Immuno)biography and somatic mutations are dynamic processes that change during aging

2. Family history shapes various gene-environment interactions (directly or indirectly).

3. Choose a statistical model to assess both the indirect effects

of parental variants and thedirect effects of inherited variants.

4. Geographical, cultural, birth cohort, and socioeconomic factors alter the interactions between genes and the environment.

5. Identify risk and protective alleles based on a socioeconomic level, geography, and birthcohort.

6. Different populations' genetic backgrounds (such as APOE) are shaped by evolutionary processes (migration and natural selection), and the genetics of longevity is population-specific.

7. Genetic analysis of each population and evolutionary medicine will aid in locating genes andpathways associated with long life in that population.

Modern technology

1. Many GWAS/gene candidate investigations of longevity found variants linked to age-relatedillnesses (such as APOE, chr9p21)

2. According to the geroscience perspective, patients with age-related diseases must be included in the study of human lifespan, and centenarians must be included as a super control group in the study of age-related diseases.

3. Age-specific genetic risk factors are important in the remodeling process.

4. Identifying the function of the genetic variations in various contexts is aided by complexallele timing and antagonistic pleiotropy dynamics.

5. GWAS revealed that genes linked to lifespan are widespread and population-specific.

6. To conduct research using controls and centenarians who share the same population geneticmakeup.

Use genome editing to assess these genes' effectsSmall-effect alleles are associated with longevity (association signals tend to be spread across most of the genome). It's possible that the GWAS threshold of 10-8 is invalid for longevity. 4. Use novel analytical techniques, such as pathway analysis or the monogenic approach Boyle et al. described for mapping cell-specific regulatory networks.

Longevity Depends on Small-Effect Alleles

The Yashin et al. GWAS study135 demonstrated the significance of including signals with P10-6 in the analysis when studying the genetics of longevity, indicating that the conventional P510-8 is probably not adequate for this characteristic. The recruitment of a large number of centenarians, particularly from the same demographic, is frequently difficult and demanding, making it impossible to apply the widely accepted cutoff in GWAS data to research on lifespan characterized by a small sample size. To find the best balance between the risk of finding false- positive signals and the potential to filter out biologically meaningful signals that fall below this cutoff, we believe that the use of statistics needs to be contextualized into the biological problem (in this example, lifespan). Yashin et al.135 used 550 k SNP data from 1173 genotyped FHS participants to test the hypothesis that multiple small-effect variants contribute to Longevity (Framingham Heart Study). They showed that the combined effect of small-effect alleles on life expectancy is strong and substantial, which helps to explain why several GWAS failed to yield a P510-8 result. The significance of assessing nonadditive (nonlinear) combined genetic effect (epistasis) to examine the genetic dose-phenotypic response link in longevity was made clear by this work. Additionally, this outcome impacts genetic computations like heritability, whose primary premise is that genetic changes in phenotypes are additive in nature.

It is necessary to develop new mathematical formulas for calculating epistasis, as well as efficient methods for reducing the large dimensionality of the data and making use of both additive and nonadditive interactions.

Small-effect alleles play a role in longevity. New types of analysis are needed to study this attribute and extract the relevant information from the genetic data. Missing heritability analyses show that the additive model alone cannot account for the full genetic contribution to the genetic dose-phenotypic response in complex characteristics. A portion of the missing heritability for human longevity should be provided by nonadditive interactions and epistasis. The ecological space idea (right) postulates that individual, time- and space-dependent gene- environment (GE) interactions are what determine longevity genetics. ID displays a centenarian in green and other non-centenarians in red, respectively.

In the study by Boyle et al, a novel approach to analyzing small- effect alleles is discussed.

They suggested a monogenic model based on the classification of core and peripheral genes. The first class of genes, according to the authors, is made up of a network of genes whose mutation results in the biggest impacts on the trait under research. In contrast, the second class of genes is made up of all the genes with no effects that appear to be significant. They discovered that several peripheral genes, which are only a few steps away from the nearest core gene in terms of the network's nodes, contribute significantly to the genetic basis of a complex trait and may influence the trait in particular tissues. According to Boyle et al.128's theory, complex features like longevity and age-related disorders are the end consequence of numerous processes involving various cell types and tissues. Therefore, it is necessary to contextualize the function of genetic variants in such situations.

Age Patterns of Allele Frequencies in GWAS Analysis Displayed Monotonic and Nonmonotonic Age Distributions

Genetic influence on survival has been demonstrated by the analysis of various allele/genotype frequencies in different age classes. This technique, known as gene frequency techniques, made it possible to categorize variants as feeble, neutral, or robust following aging trends. The gene frequency technique is predicated on two key premises: (1) Allele frequencies are the same throughout all birth cohorts taken into account, and (2) genotype-specific mortality is constant across cohorts of births. This strategy was used in two investigations. First, allele frequency may change with age according to linear trends (monotonic) or nonmonotonic patterns (typically U-shaped patterns or constant until a certain age and then linear), where allele frequency decreases until a certain age but then increases to reflect trade-offs in their impact at young and old ages.

Gene frequency approaches. Different ages have different allele/genotype frequencies. This method identified linear trends (monotonic) or nonmonotonic patterns (typically U-shaped patterns or constant until a certain age and then linear) of allele frequencies if initial allele frequencies in all birth cohorts are identical and if mortalities for genotypes do not depend on the birth cohorts. The trade-off between the impacts at young and old ages may be reflected in these trajectories.

It has been hypothesized that nonmonotonic patterns reflect genetic variations whose effect on mortality risk shifts with aging, from harmful to helpful (or vice versa).

Such trajectories add to the complexity of the research of longevity genetics since they show how an allele's impact changes depending on the internal environment as individuals age, from the youngest to the oldest.

This characteristic, referred to as complicated allele timing by De Benedictis and Franceschi, highlights the possibility that age-specific genetic hazards or protective factors exist. It is critical to distinguish between antagonistic pleiotropy and allele timing. The antagonistic pleiotropy theory states that the same allele can affect opposing qualities (such fertility or traits linked to disease) later on, during a different stage of life, in addition to the likelihood of surviving at young/adult age. Infection resistance or high fertility, for instance, may be conferred by an allele early in life. Still, the same allele may be detrimental to survival later in life. Instead, the adaptive remodeling of cellular and molecular systems that occurs throughout a lifetime is connected to the allele timing. The remodeling theory of aging states that2,143 the same allele can have various impacts on survival depending on how it functions (for example, how its genes are expressed) in the internal milieu, which alters with aging. As the effect is on the same features, this situation has no pleiotropy.

KLOTHO, a gene for aging linked to low levels of high-density lipoprotein and a decreased risk of cardiovascular disease, and LPA (lipoprotein A) genes are two examples of genes whose variations exhibit a U-shape pattern.

A Different Approach to Parental Lifespan in GWAS Studies

The ability to explore the genetics of the parental life expectancy phenotype was made possible By the availability of GWAS data in large population cohorts and the parent's age of death data

Geographical dispersion nowadays

In Europe, APOE-e4 showed a decline (from 20% in North Europe to 6/7% in Southern Europe).

A sort of U-shaped latitudinal trajectory is followed by the e4 allele in human populations, with high frequencies (up to 40%–50% of the population) in equatorial and high latitudes and low frequencies in middle latitudes.

» connection to physiological characteristics

» Regulation of synthesis and conversion of lipids

» The gene APOE-e4 is linked to elevated cholesterol.

» removing lipoproteins

» It is expressed in various organs, including the liver, adipose tissue, nervous system, andmacrophages.

» Mean luteal progesterone levels were substantially more significant in women with theAPOE-e4 allele than in those with other genotypes, indicating higher potential fertility.

» Mice carrying APOE-e4 are more susceptible to cognitive impairment from a diet low inomega-3 fatty acids.

» In APOE-e4 carriers, high levels of physical exercise lower illness chances.

» Transgenic mice harboring human versions of these proteins indicate that mice withapoE4 have impaired spatial memory, but mice with apoE3 do not.

» participation in unhealthy traits

» Alzheimer's disease (AD) and cardiovascular disorders are linked to APOE-e4.

» AD onset is later in APOE-e3 or APOE-e2 carriers than in APOE-e4 carriers.

» Longevity

» In numerous research and meta-analyses on human longevity, APOE-e4 is inverselycorrelated with longevity.

» These APOE gene variations are a part of the LD block that contains the APOE, TOMM40,and APOC1 genes.

» Apolipoprotein E is known as APOE.

Numerous studies have linked longevity to genetic variation in the IGF-1 pathway. One of the most consistently observed genetic predictors of lifespan in a range of model organisms is the IGF-1 gene family and associated genes. A wide range of activities connected to metabolic control and energy management involves the IGF-1 pathway. There is evidence that IGF-1 levelsare much lower in centenarians193 and that there is a link between increased IGF-1 levels in the blood and all-cause mortality, but not CVD events. In a study on Italian centenarians

Conducted in 2003, Bonafè et al.195 revealed a link between an SNP in the IGF-1R gene and low plasma levels of IGF-1. They also discovered that the allele responsible for the low IGF-1 levels was over-represented in centenarians. In 2008, Suh et al. sequenced the IGF-1R gene in a cohort of Ashkenazi Jewish centenarians. They discovered that these individuals were enriched in genetic variations that could lower the effectiveness of IGF-1R, resulting in the form of IGF-1 resistance. The IGF-1R rs2229765 polymorphism improves longevity in male carriers of the homozygous A allele, according to a 2011 study on an Italian cohort of people >85 years old.

The genetic variability of FOXO3, a transcription factor that inhibits the IGF-1 pathway, is one of the most reliable heritable factors associated with human longevity. According to sequencing studies, this gene's alleles associated with lifespan are found in the 3' regions.

In a study by Flachsbart et al., the author's combined candidate gene sequencing with SNP genotyping and found variations associated with lifespan in 3 North European populations, namely France, Germany, and Denmark. Mainly, two variants—rs4946935 and rs12206094— were found, one of which (rs4946935) has already been identified as a longevity gene. The results of functional validation of these two noncoding variants demonstrate that the longevity- associated allele enhances the gene's expression. In addition, the authors investigated the genetic relationship between circulating levels of IGF-1 and IGF-binding protein 3's thorough meta-analysis of 30 884 people of European ancestry. By using an innovative method, the scientists could prove a strong correlation between the circulating IGF-1 levels and the FOXO3 gene variant rs2153960. Several loci involved in the growth hormone pathway also appeared, indicating notable connections for the IGF-1, IGFBP3, IGFALS, GHSRASXL2, and CESLSR2. Many discovered variations were also linked to longevity and elderly health features. According to functional investigations, human cells may include an HSF1-FOXO3 axis implicated in stress response. Through chromatin looping, 46 additional genes on chromosome 6 joined forces with FOXO3 to establish an aging hu

CHAPTER 12

COEVOLUTION OF THE NUCLEAR
GENOME AND THE GUTMICROBIOTA
IN LONGEVITY

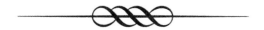

The number of studies on gut microbiota (GM) has grown significantly over the past few decades. The findings indicated that GM's composition significantly impacts age-related disorders, including CVD.

An Evolutionary Perspective on Microbiotas

It is vital to use models drawn from theoretical ecology to explain and predict the evolution of the GM ecosystem, which is a sophisticated ecosystem sensitive to environmental stimuli, host genetics, and physiological status (e.g., diet, age, among others).

A viewpoint by Foster et al. suggested that the broad holobiont concept might be misleading if applied sloppily to the host-microbiota coevolution analysis because it steers evolutionary thinking toward a conceptualization where host and microbiota would act given common interests. Instead, each microbial species and the host are autonomous evolutionary objects that respond to selective pressures and evolve following Darwinian dynamics. According to this

CHAPTER 13

WHY DO CELLS AGE?

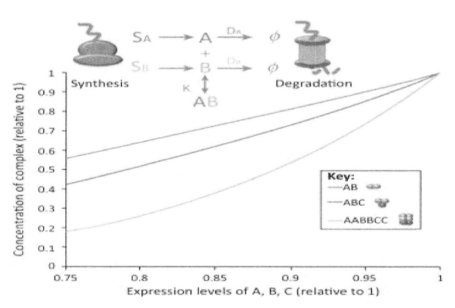

Trends in Cell Biology

Aging, physiological changes occur gradually over time and result in senescence in an organism or a loss in biological processes and an organism's capacity to respond to metabolic stress.

With time, aging occurs in a cell, an organ, or the entire organism. Any living thing engages in it throughout its adult existence. Gerontology, the study of aging, is committed to understanding and managing every element that contributes to the impermanence of individual existence. It covers a far broader spectrum of occurrences rather than focusing solely on debility, which dominates the human experience. Every species has a life history in which the length of the individual life span is correctly correlated with the size of the reproductive life span, the mode of reproduction, and the progression of development. Both evolutionary biology and gerontology are relevant to the evolution of these partnerships. It's crucial to distinguish between the unintentional organismic processes of sickness and injury resulting in mortality and the merely physicochemical processes of aging.

Therefore, gerontology can be summed up as the study of the three characteristics of longevity, aging, and death from both an evolutionary and an individual (ontogenetic) perspective. The length of an organism's life is its longevity. Aging is an organism's gradual or progressive alteration that raises the risk of disease, debility, and death. These aging-related characteristics are referred to as senescence.

The survivorship curve and the age-specific death rate, or the Gompertz function, are two actuarial functions that describe the viability (ability to survive) of a population. The relationship between actuarial functions and variables, including aging traits, constitutional Vigor, physical factors, food, and exposure to pathogens, is complicated. But as indicators of aging and the impact of hereditary or environmental factors, there is no alternative for them.

The age-specific death rate is the most useful actuarial function for aging process research. Benjamin Gompertz, an English actuary, made the initial observation that the death rate rises geometrically, or by a fixed ratio in succeeding intervals of similar ages, in 1825. Therefore, when death rates are plotted on a logarithmic (ratio) scale, a straight line, known as the Gompertz function, results. With some notable exceptions, such as viral diseases and diseases caused by immune system disruptions, the incidence of many diseases and disabilities rises in the same geometric fashion as the mortality rate. Even related species can differ greatly in the relative incidence of the primary causes of mortality, even though the life tables of most species are very similar in shape.

Life expectancy for people in industrialized nations has dramatically increased. In fact, those nations' life expectancies at the start of the 20th century ranged from 30 to 45 years. Life expectancy rose to an average of 67 years at the end of the century, mainly due to advancements in diet, health care, and living standards. According to demographic predictions made in the early 21st century, men and women who follow the healthiest living patterns will live longer. The fastest-growing population group in the United States in the first decade of the twenty-first century was centenarians or people who live to be 100 or older.

What results in cell aging?

Recent research has revealed an unanticipated function for a protein linked to early aging. Furthermore, they demonstrated how it controls cellular senescence to support their claim that its absence causes normal aging.

Our lives will inevitably include aging. However, aging populations present problems for public health.

Research predicts that there will be around 71 million Americans aged 65 and older in the following ten years.

But what indeed occurs as we become older? Numerous theories are under development by scientists and trusted Sources.

Cockayne syndrome B (CSB), a protein implicated in repairing damaged DNA and early aging, has been the subject of research at the Institute Pasteur in Paris, France.

The team explains in a paper published in the Nature Communications Trusted Source that as cells age, their normal production of this protein decreases, triggering cellular senescence.

Seniority and senescence

The biological process of senescence restricts a cell's capacity to divide. It often occurs when a cell sustains significant damage from stress-related events.

While still living, senescent cells cannot divide. Instead, it secretes signaling chemicals to communicate with other cells and has a busy metabolism. This may be advantageous when a wound is healing or harmful, as in the case of chronic inflammation.

The CSB protein is mutated in individuals with Cockayne syndrome, which causes early aging and other symptoms.

To determine whether CSB may be a factor in promoting typical aging, senior research author Miria Ricchetti and her associates conducted the investigation.

preventing senility

Why do mitochondria exist?

➤ Mitochondria are frequently referred to as the "powerhouses" of the cell. They aid in transforming the energy that comes from food into energy that the cell can use. But mitochondria are engaged in more than just the creation of energy.

➤ Mitochondria, found in almost every type of human cell, are essential to our life. Most of our adenosine triphosphate (ATP), the cell's energy currency, is produced by them.

➤ Apoptosis, also known as cell death, and communicating between cells are two more actions that mitochondria do.

➤ This article will examine mitochondria, describe how they appear, and explain what occurs when they cease functioning properly.

The form of the mitochondria

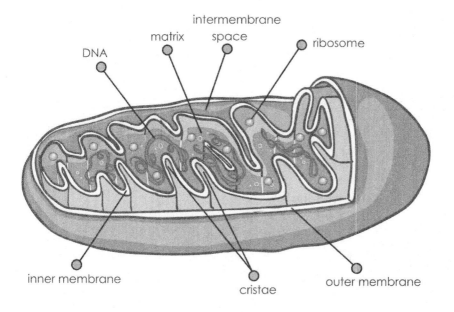

» The size of mitochondria, which is frequently between 0.75 and 3 micrometers, makes them difficult to see under a microscope unless labeled.

» They have two membranes, an outer and an inner one, in contrast to other organelles,which are tiny organs within the cell. Different membranes serve various purposes.

» Each of the several compartments or sections that make up mitochondria performs aspecific function.

» The following are some of the major regions:

» Small molecules can effortlessly pass through the outer membrane. Porins, a class of proteins found in this outer layer, provide channels through which other proteins can pass. Many enzymes with diverse functions are also present in the outer membrane.

» The space between the inner and outer membranes is known as the intermembranespace.

» The inner membrane is where proteins with various functions are stored. The innermembrane is impervious to most molecules because it lacks porins. Only particular membrane transporters can transport molecules through the inner membrane. Themajority of ATP is produced in the inner membrane.

Cristae: These are the inner membrane's folds. They expand the membrane's surface area, expanding the amount of room accessible for chemical processes.

The matrix is the region located inside the inner membrane. It has numerous enzymes and makes a major contribution to ATP synthesis. This is where mitochondrial DNA is kept (see below).

The quantity of mitochondria varies between different types of cells. For instance, liver cells can have more than 2,000, but mature red blood cells have zero. Mitochondria are more prevalent in cells that require a lot of energy. For example, mitochondria occupy about 40% of the cytoplasm in cardiac muscle cells.

Despite being represented as oval-shaped organelles, mitochondria regularly divide (fission) and join together (fusion) (fusion). As a result, these organelles are genuinely connected by dynamic networks.

Furthermore, the mitochondria in sperm cells are coiled in the midpiece and supply energy for tail motion.

DNA from mitochondria

Although most of our DNA is stored in each cell's nucleus, mitochondria also contain their own DNA. It's interesting to note that mtDNA resembles bacterial DNA more.

» Over 37 genes, the mtDNA stores the blueprints for several proteins and other pieces ofcellular machinery.

» 3.3 billion base pairs comprise the human genome, which is kept in the cell nuclei,whereas less than 17,000 base pairs make up mtDNA.

» A child's DNA is divided in half during reproduction, with the other half coming from themother. However, the mother is always where the child gets their mtDNA from. As a result, mtDNA has been particularly effective in tracking genetic lines.

For instance, mtDNA tests have determined that humans may have sprung from a common ancestor, mitochondrial Eve, who originated in Africa very recently, perhaps 200,000 years ago, trusted Source.

Why do mitochondria function?

Although energy production is the most well-known function of mitochondria, they also perform other crucial functions.

In actuality, only roughly 3% of the genes required to create a mitochondrion are found in its energy-generating machinery. Instead, most of them are engaged in additional tasks unique to the cell type in which they are present.

We discuss a few of the functions of the mitochondria below:

Generating energy

Because it drives metabolic processes, ATP, a complex organic molecule in all living things, is frequently referred to as the molecular equivalent of money. Most ATP is created in mitochondria through a series of processes called the Krebs or citric acid cycle.

The inner membrane's folds or cristae are where most energy is produced.

Chemical energy from the food we eat is transformed by mitochondria into an energy source that the cell can utilize. The term for this procedure is oxidative phosphorylation.

During the Krebs cycle, the substance NADH is created. Enzymes included in the cristaeuse NADH to create ATP. Chemical bonds serve as energy reservoirs in ATP molecules. The energy can be put to use after these chemical bonds are broken.

Cells die

Apoptosis, another name for cell death, is a necessary aspect of life. Cells are removed and destroyed when they get older or break. Mitochondria have a role in cell death decision-making.

Cytochrome C, released by mitochondria, activates caspase, one of the main enzymes responsible for cell death during apoptosis.

As a breakdown in normal apoptosis occurs in certain disorders, such as cancer, mitochondria are assumed to be involved in the sickness.

Preserving Calcium

Numerous biological activities require Calcium to function. For instance, reintroducing Calcium into a cell might cause the release of hormones from endocrine cells or neurotransmitters from nerve cells. , Calcium is also essential for several processes like blood coagulation, fertilization, and muscle function.

Calcium is tightly regulated by the cell because it is so important. Mitochondria play a role in swiftly collecting calcium ions and storing them until they are required Calcium also controls cellular metabolism, steroid production, and hormone communication in the cell dependable Source

Creation of heat

We shudder to stay warm when we are cold. However, there are additional ways for the body to produce heat, one of which is utilizing a tissue known as brown fat.

Mitochondria are capable of producing heat via a process known as proton leak. Non-shivering thermogenesis is the term for this. When we are young and more prone to colds, brown fat is in the highest concentrations. As we become older, levels gradually decline.

Molecular illness

Mitochondrial DNA is more prone to damage than the rest of the genome, This is because ATP production produces free radicals, which can harm DNA Also, mitochondria lack the same defense systems as the cell's nucleus.

However, the bulk of mitochondrial disorders is brought on by changes in nuclear DNA that impact mitochondrial products. Both spontaneous and hereditary mutations are possible.

The cell they are in runs out of energy when the mitochondria cease working. Consequently, the symptoms can vary greatly depending on the type of cell. Cells that require the most energy, such as nerve and heart muscle cells, are typically affected by defective mitochondria.

From the United Mitochondrial Disease Foundation, the following passage:

"There are hundreds of different mitochondrial illnesses because mitochondria carry out various tasks in various organs. It is a feature of mitochondrial disorders that similar mtDNA mutations may not create identical diseases because of the complicated interplay between the hundreds of genes and cells that must work together to keep our metabolic machinery working smoothly.

Genocopies are diseases that exhibit various symptoms yet result from the same mutation.

On the other hand, diseases are referred to as phenocopies when they share the same symptoms but are brought on by mutations in separate genes. Leigh syndrome is an illustration of a phenocopy that is brought on by numerous distinct mutations.

Despite the wide variety of symptoms associated with mitochondrial diseases, they may include:

» weakness and a loss of muscle coordination
» issues with hearing or vision learning difficulties
» renal, liver, or cardiac disease
» abdominal discomfort
» neurological conditions, such as dementia

The following disorders are thought to also entail some degree of mitochondrialdysfunction:

» Parkinson's disease
» Alzheimer's disease
» bipolar disorder
» schizophrenia
» chronic fatigue syndrome
» Huntington's disease
» diabetes
» autism

Aging and mitochondria

Researchers have looked at the connection between aging and mitochondrial malfunction. There are numerous ideas concerning aging. Over the past ten years, the mitochondrial free radical theory of aging has gained popularity.

Reactive oxygen species (ROS), according to the notion, are created in mitochondria as a consequence of energy synthesis. These incredibly charged particles harm proteins, lipids, and DNA.

The functioning components of mitochondria are harmed as a result of ROS damage. More ROS are formed when the mitochondria can no longer perform as well, which worsens the damage.

Although there have been links between mitochondrial activity and aging, not all researchers have come to the same findings. Their precise part in aging is still a mystery.

Briefly said, mitochondria are arguably the most well-known organelle. And while though they are frequently described as the center of the cell, they also perform a variety of lesser-known functions. The daily operations of our cells rely heavily on mitochondria, which do everything from store calcium to produce heat.

Aging biologically

Most people will live long enough to age. But unfortunately, more and more people are negatively impacted by aging. Even if the process cannot be avoided, it is crucial to comprehend it. As physiotherapists, we may be able to help maintain or promote greater health and wellness as a person ages by treating and easing the symptoms of common aging-related diseases.

It was believed that the maximum life span—the biological limit of life in an ideal environment—was not prone to change since aging was regarded as a non-adaptive process influenced by genetic features. However, researchers Alexis Carrel conducted a series of erroneous experiments in the early 1900s that showed that higher creatures' (chickens') cells might divide continuously in an ideal environment, which led people to speculate that human cells might be capable of immortality. By determining the maximum number of divisions, a human cell may undergo in culture (known as the Hayflick limit), Leonard Hayflick refuted this hypothesis in the 1960s, setting our maximum life span at about 115 years. Life expectancy is key to understanding the fundamental biological elements that contribute to aging since it determines how long an individual will live before succumbing to the effects of biological aging.

No single hypothesis can adequately describe the process of aging, and there are numerous explanations about the mechanisms underlying age-related changes that are mutually exclusive. According to a literature review, centenarians age in a healthy way since age-related illnesses and physiological decline are delayed in this population. The review talks about how essential a genetic factor is for longevity. The specialists claim that understanding the biology of centenarians can help us understand how to encourage healthy aging in a larger population.

Planned aging and damage or error theories are the two main categories of contemporary biological explanations of human aging.

According to the damage or error hypotheses, aging is brought on by environmental assaults on living things that accumulate over time at different levels. In contrast, programmed theories contend that aging occurs according to a biological timetable (regulated by changes in gene expression that affect the systems responsible for maintenance, repair, and defense responses).

These two theories are also referred to as non-programmed aging theories based on evolutionary concepts (where aging is thought to be the result of an organism's inability to more successfully fight off natural deteriorative processes) and programmed aging theories (which hold that aging is ultimately the result of a biological mechanism or program that purposely causes or allows deterioration and death to obtain a direct evolutionary benefit obtained

CHAPTER 14

AGING THEORIES

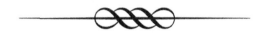

Three subcategories of the planned theory and four subcategories of the damage or mistake theory are highlighted by Jim in his overview of contemporary theories of aging. He also connects to how these might be seen in aging populations.

Ageing Biological Theories

The Theory of Programs

1. Programmed Longevity views aging as the outcome of a series of gene activations and suppressions, with senescence defined as the point at which age-related deficiencies become apparent.

2. The endocrine theory holds that biological clocks regulate the rate of aging through hormones.

3. The Immunological Theory contends that as we age, our immune systems become more susceptible to infectious diseases, which accelerates the aging process and causes us to die.

The Theory of Damage or Error

1. The wear-and-tear theory states that important components deteriorate as our cells andtissues age.

2. The rate of living theory contends that an organism's life span is shortened by a higher rateof oxygen basal metabolism.

3. The aggregation of cross-linked proteins harms cells and tissues, slows down body functions, and causes aging, according to the cross-linking theory.

4. The free radical's theory contends that superoxide and other free radicals destroy the macromolecular building blocks of cells, accumulating damage that prevents cells and organs from functioning.

Additional Theories

An alternative perspective is offered by Trindade et al. They claim that to comprehend the evolution of aging, we must comprehend the environment-dependent balance between the benefits and drawbacks of an extended lifespan in gene spreading. In their fitness-based paradigm, these researchers have divided the various ideas into four fundamental categories: secondary (helpful), maladaptive (neutral), aided death (harmful), and senemorphic aging (varying between beneficial to detrimental).

The following is an overview of some of the aging-related theories that are more frequently discussed:

» Theory of Disengagement
» Refers to an inescapable process in which many of a person's interactions with otherpeople in society are severed & those that remain are changed.

- » Withdrawal might be partial or complete and can be started by society or the elderly.
- » Elderly folks have been seen to be less engaged in life than younger adults.
- » People grow more removed from society as they get older and form new connectionswith it.
- » There is evidence that older individuals in America are forced to retreat by society,whether or not they like to.
- » Some claim that this hypothesis fails to consider the significant proportion of elderlypeople who remain active in society.
- » This idea is acknowledged as the first official theory that made an effort to explain theaging process.

Another idea that explains the psychosocial aging process is Activity Theory

According to activity theory, constant social interaction is crucial.

According to this hypothesis, a person's self-concept is correlated with the roles they actively maintain. For example, retiring may not be as detrimental if a person actively maintains other responsibilities, including familial, recreational, volunteer, and community duties.

A person must fill in for duties lost as they get older to keep a positive sense of self. So, the type of activity does crucial, according to research, just as it does for younger people.

The Neuroendocrine Theory, initially put forth by Dr. Ward Dean and Professor Vladimir Dilman, elaborates on wear and tear by concentrating on the neuroendocrine system.

The hypothalamus, a brain-based gland about the size of a walnut, controls the release of hormones through a complex network of biochemicals in this system.

The hypothalamus regulates several chain reactions that tell other glands and organs when and how to release hormones, among other things. Regarding total hormonal activity, the hypothalamus also reacts to body hormone levels. However, as we age, the hypothalamus loses its ability to precisely regulate, and the receptors that take in certain hormones become less sensitive. As a result, as we age, several hormones become less secreted and less efficient (compared to one another). This is because the receptors in our bodies slow down. grading

The free-radical hypothesis

At the University of Nebraska in 1956, Dr. Denham Harman created the now-famous theory of aging. Any molecule with an unoccupied electron is referred to as a free radical. Because of this, it reacts negatively with other healthy molecules.

The extra electron in the free radical molecule results in an additional negative charge. To steal electrons, this imbalanced energy causes the free radical to bond to another balanced molecule. By doing this, the balanced molecule goes out of equilibrium and turns into a free radical.

It is well known that diet, way of life, drugs (including alcohol and tobacco), radiation, etc., all speed up the body's generation of free radicals.

The Ageing Membrane Theory

Imre Zs.-Nagy of Debrechen University in Hungary is the person who originally introduced the membrane hypothesis of aging. This idea holds that the cell's ability to transport chemicals, heat and electrical processes becomes impaired as it ages.

The lipid content of the cell membrane decreases with age (less watery and more solid). This makes it more difficult to carry out routine tasks, and in particular, there is a poisonous buildup.

The Theory of Decline

In every cell of every organ, there are organelles called mitochondria that produce energy. They do this in the many energy cycles that involve nutrients like Acetyl-L-Carnitine, CoQ10 (Idebenone), NADH, certain B vitamins, and others. Their main task is to produce adenosine triphosphate (ATP).

The mitochondria must be strengthened and protected to stop and slow down aging. The nutrients above can improve performance, as can ATP supplements themselves.

The Theory of Cross-Linking

The Glycosylation Theory of Aging is another name for the Cross-Linking Theory of Aging. According to this view, numerous issues are brought on by binding glucose (simple sugars) to protein. This process takes place when oxygen is present.

Once this binding has occurred, the protein is impaired and can no longer function as effectively. In addition, longer life will increase the likelihood of oxygen interacting with glucose and protein, and known cross-linking problems include senile cataracts and the development of rough, leathery, and yellow skin.

Aging and psychological theories

Age-related notions have their roots in psychological theories. These ideas focus on an individual's conduct, outlook on life, and personality changes or ego development as they relate to aging. The psychological theories of aging place a strong emphasis on the adjustments in mental functions, feelings, attitudes, and motivation due to physical, social, or environmental demands. This capacity for adaptation is thought to be influenced by social status changes, changes in relationships as people age, and role changes.

Theory of Human Needs

This hypothesis, which Maslow developed in 1954, emphasizes that as people age, their needs become more important in driving their behavior. These requirements include physical security and safety, a sense of love and belonging, self-worth, and actualization.

Physical needs: There is a strong need to receive food, drink, and shelter, and behaviors assure that these needs are met. Most people don't need assistance with this, but some people, especially those with cognitive impairments, might. Safety and Security: This need has both immediate and long-term effects, such as the desire to avoid dangerous areas and work toward creating a safer society. In contrast to food, water, and shelter, these needs are more ethereal, and pursuing them further necessitates some imaginative thinking. While innate responses to hunger, thirst, and the elements exist, recognizing and responding to veiled dangers can be challenging. The kind of training associated with these needs is also very different from those associated with physical wants because the need for security is frequently only noticed when it is threatened or lost.

In contrast, the rewards of getting food are immediate and visceral. Belonging and Love: The likelihood of belonging is greatly increased by the ability to communicate via phone, email, or social networking sites. Families of patients with cognitive impairments frequently look for ways to stay "virtually" in touch across space and time to satisfy their loved ones' needs for affection and belonging. Even patients with significant cognitive impairments appreciate social interaction because it offers immediate and easy rewards like acceptance and affection. Esteem requirements: People desire to be respected and believed in. This comprises completing tasks that a person values to earn money. Limiting someone's access to such activities can make them feel less confident. Self-actualization needs: The highest degrees of human desires are loyalty to one's nature and the pursuit of self-fulfillment through creativity. Self-actualization can be accomplished by doing activities that make you feel completely alive or by taking part in something with a higher purpose after all previous levels of need have been satisfied. This need can be satisfied in various ways, including through artistic pursuits, professional careers, charitable work, community service, and hobbies, as well as mature and tolerant interpersonal interactions and communication styles.

Theory of Individualism

Jung proposed in 1960 that our ego and self-identity, both individually and collectively unconscious, are the building blocks of our personality, which develops over time. Personal unconsciousness is a private mood or experience related to significant persons or life events.

Theory of Life-Course (Lifespan Development)

created in the 1980s by behavioral psychologists who decided to use the concept of "life cycle" instead of personality development as the foundation for aging understanding. According to this view, the stages of life may be predicted and are produced by objectives, relationships, and personal values. The connection between the individual and society is the main theme of this ideology.

Baltes proposed the Selective Optimization and Compensation Theory in 1987. He felt that through a process of selection, optimization, and compensation, humans eventually learn to deal with the unique losses associated with age. As people mature, adaptation is carried out through choosing more fulfilling vocations. Baltes thinks carefully chosen optimization in conjunction with compensation is a positive coping mechanism that promotes successful aging.

Describe epigenetics

Your environment and behaviors, such as what you eat and how active you are, are just as crucial to your health as your genes. Epigenetics studies how environmental factors and behavior can alter how your genes function. While epigenetic alterations are reversible and do not alter your DNA sequence like genetic changes, they can alter how your body interprets a DNA sequence.

The frequency or timing of protein synthesis from your genes' instructions is called gene expression. While epigenetic alterations impact gene expression to switch genes "on" and "off," genetic modifications can modify which proteins are produced. It is simple to show how your genes, behaviors, and environment are related since your environment and activities, such as nutrition and exercise, can cause epigenetic alterations.

CHAPTER 15

THE MECHANISM OF EPIGENETIC

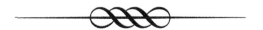

Different epigenetic modifications have an impact on gene expression. Various epigenetic modifications include:

Methylation of DNA

When DNA is methylated, a chemical group is added. This group is typically introduced to particular regions of DNA, which prevents proteins from attaching to DNA and "reading" genes. Demethylation, a procedure, can be used to get rid of this chemical group. Genes are typically "turned off" by methylation and "turned on" by demethylation.

Histone alteration

Histone proteins are encircled by DNA. Proteins that "read" the gene cannot reach DNA securely encased by histones. While some genes are "off" because they are wrapped around histones, others are "on" because they are not. Histones can have chemical groups added or deleted, which alters whether a gene is wrapped or unwrapped (or "on" or "off").

RNA with no codons

Coding and non-coding RNA are produced using instructions found in your DNA. Proteins are created using coding RNA. By joining with specific proteins and coding RNA to break down the coding RNA, which prevents it from being utilized to produce proteins, non-coding RNA regulates gene expression. To "on" or "off" genes, non-coding RNA may also enlist proteins to change histones.

Infections

Your immune system might be weakened by germs by altering your epigenetics. The germ can survive as a result.

Example: Tuberculosis-causing mycobacterium

Tuberculosis is brought on by Mycobacterium tuberculosis. This is because some of your immune cells may experience histone modifications due to infections with certain pathogens, which turn the IL-12B gene "off." When the IL-12B gene is "turned off," the immune system is compromised and Mycobacterium tuberculosis has a higher likelihood of survival.

Cancer

Several mutations increase your risk of getting cancer. The chance of developing cancer is increased by some epigenetic modifications. For instance, getting breast and other cancers increases your risk if you have a mutation in the BRCA1 gene that stops it from functioning normally. Similar to this, more DNA methylation increases the chance of developing breast and other cancers by lowering the expression of the BRCA1 gene. Although some genes in cancer cells have more DNA methylation than in healthy cells, overall DNA methylation levels in cancer cells are lower than in healthy cells. Even cancers that appear to be the same type can differ in their DNA methylation patterns. Epigenetics can be used to identify the sort of cancer a person has or to locate malignancies that were difficult to find earlier. Cancers need to be validated with other screening tests since epigenetics alone cannot identify cancer.

For instance, colorectal cancer:

The expression of certain genes is impacted by abnormal DNA methylation at regions close to these genes in colorectal cancers. Stool samples are sometimes used in commercial colorectal cancer screening tests to check for abnormal DNA methylation levels at one or more of these DNA regions. It is crucial to understand that a colonoscopy test is required to complete the screening process if the test result is positive or abnormal.

Eating Well While Pregnant:

The epigenetic makeup of the unborn child can be altered by the surroundings and actions of the pregnant woman, such as whether or not she consumes a healthy diet. Some of these alterations might increase the child's risk of contracting specific diseases and last for decades.

Using the Dutch Winter Famine as an example (1944-1945)

Those whose mothers carried them during the famine had a higher risk of developing heart disease, schizophrenia, and type 2 diabetes (6). Researchers examined methylation levels in individuals whose mothers carried them during the famine about 60 years after it ended. These people displayed increased methylation at some genes compared to their siblings who were not starved before birth. On the other hand, they reduced the methylation of other genes. These changes in methylation may help explain why these people had an increased chance of contracting particular diseases later in life.

Chapter 16

Epigenetic clock:
A Hopeful Age-Reflection Mirror

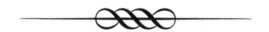

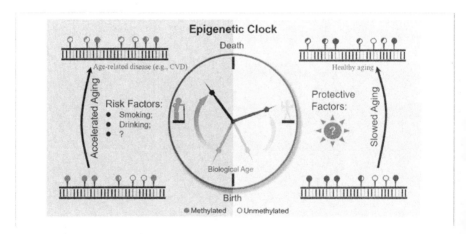

Aging according to the epigenetic clock

A novel, comprehensive theory of aging and the emergence of complex diseases was put forth in 2010. It included both epigenetic and conventional theories of aging.

Horvath and Raj expanded on this idea by putting forth an epigenetic clock theory of aging that adheres to the following principles:

Biological aging is an unexpected byproduct of maintenance and developmental systems, whose molecular traces give rise to DNA methylation age estimators

The precise mechanisms relating internal alterations (resulting in a loss of cellular identity) and minor changes in cell composition, such as fully functional somatic stem cells, to the deterioration in tissue function, are presumably related to both.

DNAm age is a molecular readout of several inherent aging processes that work in concert with other separate root causes of aging to impair tissue function.

The rationale behind biological clocks

Since age is a fundamental property of most organisms, biological aging clocks and biomarkers of aging are anticipated to find numerous applications in biological study. The use of precise biological age measurements (aging clocks) could be beneficial for

> » evaluating the truth of different biological aging theories,
> » identifying cancer subtypes and detecting a variety of age-related illnesses,
> » detecting the onset of several diseases and providing a prognosis,
> » acting as proxies for evaluating therapeutic therapies, such as methods of rejuvenation,
> » investigating cell differentiation and developmental biology,
> » forensic uses, such as determining a suspect's age from the blood left at a crime scene.

In general, it is anticipated that biological clocks will help research what causes aging and what can be done to prevent it. However, they cannot capture the effects of interventions that act at a specific point in time, such as lowering mortality across all ages, which corresponds to the intercept of the Gompertz curve. Instead, they can only be used to measure the effects of Interventions that change the rate of future aging or the slope of the Gompertz curve by which mortality increases with age.

Horvath's clock characteristics

The clock is a technique for estimating age based on 353 epigenetic DNA markers. The CpG dinucleotide methylation in DNA is measured by the 353 markers. DNA methylation age, also known as estimated age or predicted age in mathematics, has the following characteristics: it is almost zero for embryonic and induced pluripotent stem cells; it correlates with the number of cell passages; it produces a highly heritable measure of age acceleration, and it applies to chimpanzee tissues (which are used as human analogs for biological testing purposes). After reaching adulthood, the epigenetic clock decreases to a constant ticking rate (linear dependency) from the high ticking rate caused by organismal growth (and accompanying cell division) (age 20). Even after correcting for known risk variables, blood DNA methylation age predicts all-cause mortality in later life. Is consistent with a wide range of causal connections, including a common cause for both. Similarly, the epigenetic clock is linked to indicators of both physical and mental health (lower abilities associated with age acceleration). It consistently underestimates age in older people.

Horvath's epigenetic clock stands out for its application to various tissues and cell types. It is possible to distinguish tissues that exhibit signs of accelerated aging brought on by disease since it allows one to compare the ages of various tissues from the same patient.

Statistical method

The fundamental strategy is to create a weighted average of the 353 clocks CpGs, which is calibrated to DNAm age. According to the calibration function, the epigenetic clock ticks quickly up to adulthood and then gradually slows down to a steady rate. Horvath regressed 21,369 CpG probes that were found on the Illumina 450K and 27K platforms and had less than 10 missing values using a penalized regression model (Elastic net regularization) using the training data sets. The term "DNAm age" refers to estimated (or "predicted") age. 353 CpGs were chosen by the elastic net predictor automatically. Of the 353 CpGs, 193 have a positive correlation with age, whereas the remaining 160 have a negative correlation. You may find R software and a free online tool at the following website.

Accuracy

The median error of estimated age is 3.6 years across a variety of tissues and cell types, albeit this increases with age.

The epigenetic clock functions well in a variety of heterogeneous tissues, including whole blood, peripheral blood mononuclear cells, cerebellar samples, occipital cortex, buccal epithelium, colon, adipose, kidney, liver, lung, saliva, uterine cervix, epidermis, and muscle, as well as in specific cell types, including CD4 T cells, CD14 monocytes, glial cells, neurons, immortalized B However, the source of the DNA has some bearing on accuracy.

CHAPTER 17

EVALUATION OF

SEVERAL BIOLOGICAL CLOCKS

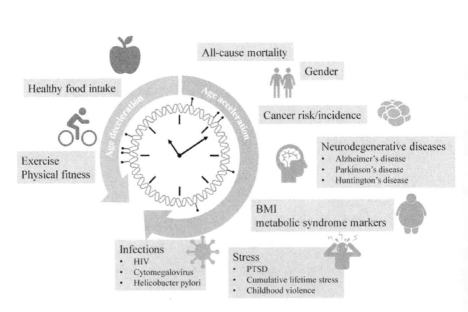

The Pearson correlation coefficient between the epigenetic clock's prediction of chronological age and chronological age is 0.96. As a result, the age correlation is very close to its highest correlation value of 1. Telomere length, p16INK4a expression levels, the INK4a/ARF locus, and microsatellite mutations are three additional biological clocks. Men and women have an r =

0.55 and 0.51 connection between chronological age and telomere length, respectively. Age chronologically and p16INK4a expression levels in T cells have an r = 0.56 association.

Uses for the Horvath clock

One can identify indices of age acceleration by comparing the projected age based on DNA methylation to chronological age. The gap between chronological and DNA methylation age is known as age acceleration. It can also be described as the leftover after DNAm age is regressed against chronological age. Because it has no relationship to chronological age, the latter measurement is appealing. A positive or negative epigenetic age acceleration number indicates that the underlying tissue ages more quickly or slowly than is typical.

Epigenetic age acceleration genetic research

Blood from older patients has a broad sense heritability (measured by Falconer's formula) of age acceleration of about 40%. However, it seems to be much higher in neonates.

The prefrontal cortex, which shows age acceleration, was observed to accelerate by 41% in older participants. In addition, genome-wide association studies (GWAS) of epigenetic age acceleration have found numerous SNPs with genome-wide significance in postmortem brain samples. Telomerase reverse transcriptase gene (TERT) locus is one of the genome-wide significant genetic loci that have been found in GWAS of age acceleration in blood. Contrary to expectations, TERT gene polymorphisms linked to greater leukocyte telomere length paradoxically confer higher blood epigenetic age acceleration.

Lifestyle elements

There are relatively sporadic connections between lifestyle factors and blood's epigenetic age acceleration.

According to cross-sectional research, reduced extrinsic epigenetic aging rates in the blood are correlated with greater education, consuming a diet high in plants and lean meats, moderate alcohol intake, physical activity, and the risks of metabolic syndrome. However, research points to a link between heavy drinking and accelerated aging of some epigenetic clocks.

The metabolic syndrome and obesity

The association between a high body mass index (BMI) and the DNA methylation ages of human blood, liver, muscle, and adipose tissue was investigated using the epigenetic clock.

For the liver, there was a discernible relationship (r = 0.42) between BMI and epigenetic age acceleration. The link between BMI and the intrinsic age acceleration of blood was weak but statistically significant (r = 0.09), according to a significantly larger study size (n = 4200 blood samples). [34] The same extensive study discovered a link between epigenetic age acceleration in blood and several metabolic syndrome biomarkers, including glucose, insulin, triglyceride, C- reactive protein, and waist-to-hip ratio. On the other hand, a lower rate of blood epigenetic aging was linked to high levels of the beneficial cholesterol HDL. With evidence that physical activity may mitigate these effects, other research points to strong associations between increased body mass index, waist-to-hip ratio, waist circumference, and accelerated epigenetic clocks.

Breast tissue in women is older than expected

In female breast tissue close to breast cancer tissue, DNAm age is older than chronological age.

This research shows that normal female breast tissue ages more quickly than other body regions since normal tissue close to other cancer types does not show a similar age acceleration impact. Similarly, it has been discovered that blood samples taken at the same time as normal breast tissue samples from cancer-free women are significantly older than the latter.

Breast cancer in women

The DNAm age of cancer-free women's blood samples was shown to be accelerated years before diagnosis in a study involving three epigenetic clocks and breast cancer risk.

Tissue with cancer exhibits both good and negative consequences of age acceleration. For most tumor types, there is no discernible correlation between age acceleration and tumor morphology (grade/stage). On average, the age acceleration of cancer tissues with mutant TP53 is less than that of cancer tissues without it. Furthermore, compared to cancer tissues with low age acceleration, those with high age acceleration typically exhibit fewer somatic mutations.

Age acceleration and numerous genetic abnormalities in cancer tissues are strongly correlated. Breast cancer DNA ages more quickly due to somatic mutations in estrogen or progesterone receptors. Age acceleration is more prevalent in colorectal cancer samples with the BRAF (V600E) mutation or promoter hypermethylation of the MLH1 mismatch repair gene. Age acceleration strongly correlates with certain H3F3A mutations in glioblastoma multiforme samples. According to one study, blood tissue's epigenetic age may predict the likelihood of developing lung cancer.

21 trisomy (Down syndrome)

The risk of numerous chronic diseases, normally linked to aging, is raised in people with Down syndrome. Trisomy 21 may cause tissues to age more quickly biologically, according to clinical signs of accelerated aging; however, there isn't many molecular data to support this theory.

Trisomy 21 dramatically lengthens the age of blood and brain tissue, according to the epigenetic clock (on average, by 6.6 years).

Neuropathology associated with Alzheimer's disease

Numerous neuropathological parameters related to Alzheimer's disease were shown to be correlated with the epigenetic age acceleration of the human prefrontal cortex.

It was also discovered to be connected to a loss in global and memory performance in people with Alzheimer's. [30] Blood's epigenetic age is related to how well seniors' brains function. Overall, these findings clearly imply that it is possible to determine the biological age of the brain using the epigenetic clock.

Slow cerebellar aging

Due to the paucity of indicators of tissue age that enable one to compare the ages of various tissues, it has been challenging to find tissues that seem to resist aging. The cerebellum ages more slowly than anticipated in a centenarian, being around 15 years younger than anticipated after applying the epigenetic clock to 30 anatomic regions from six centenarians and younger participants. This discovery may help explain why, compared to other brain regions, the cerebellum shows fewer neuropathological signs of aging-related dementias. Brain areas and cells appear to be nearly the same age in persons younger than 70. The cerebellum's epigenetic age has been linked to several SNPs and genes.

Alzheimer's disease

Huntington's disease has accelerated multiple human brain regions' epigenetic aging rates Centenarians age more gradually.

Centenarians are younger (8.6 years) than would be predicted based on their chronological age. In comparison, the progeny of semi-supercentenarians (subjects who reached an age of 105– 109 years) have younger epigenetic ages than age-matched controls (age difference = 5.1 years in the blood).

Having HIV

Clinical signs of accelerated aging are linked to Human Immunodeficiency Virus-1 (HIV) infection, as shown by the increased prevalence and variety of age-related disorders at young ages. However, it has proven challenging to identify a molecular effect of accelerated aging. HIV-1 infection caused a significant age acceleration effect in brain tissue (7.4 years) and blood tissue (5.2 years), according to an epigenetic clock analysis of human DNA from HIV+ individuals and controls. These findings align with a study that discovered a 5-year age increase in the blood of HIV patients and a significant HLA locus effect.

Parkinson's condition

According to a large-scale study, the granulocyte ratio of people with Parkinson's disease shows (very mild) signs of accelerated aging.

Syndrome X is a developmental condition

Children with syndrome X, a relatively unusual condition, age from infancy to maturity with the appearance of having permanent toddler-like traits. These kids appear to be toddlers or, at most, preschoolers because of their markedly delayed physical development. According to an epigenetic clock analysis, blood samples from syndrome X sufferers are not older than anticipated.

Epigenetic aging is accelerated by menopause.

The results below imply that menopause-related female hormone loss speeds up the blood's epigenetic aging process and may also affect other tissues.

First, early menopause has been linked to a higher rate of blood's epigenetic age acceleration.

Second, surgical menopause brought on by bilateral oophorectomy is linked to blood and salivary epigenetic age acceleration. Third, a negative age acceleration of buccal cells is linked to menopausal hormone therapy, which lessens hormonal loss (but not blood cells). Fourth, epigenetic age acceleration in the blood is linked to genetic markers connected to early menopause.

Epigenetic versus cellular senescence aging

The nature and function of senescent cells are perplexing features of biological aging. It is unknown how the three main types of cellular senescence—replicative senescence, oncogene- induced senescence, and DNA damage-induced senescence—are connected to epigenetic aging or if they are distinct descriptions of the same phenomena brought on by various sources.

Senescence brought on by DNA damage was not observed to be accompanied by epigenetic aging of primary cells, even though replicative senescence (RS) and oncogene-induced senescence (OIS) both activate the cellular DNA damage response system. These findings demonstrate the distinction between cellular senescence and epigenetic aging. The fact that telomerase-immortalized cells continued to age following the epigenetic clock despite not being exposed to any senescence-inducing or DNA-damaging substances supports the idea that epigenetic aging is unrelated to telomeres, cellular senescence, or the DNA damage response pathway. Even though senescent cells contribute to the physical expression of organism aging, as revealed by Baker et al., who found that removing senescent cells slowed down aging, senescence and cellular aging can be decoupled from one another.

However, according to the epigenetic clock analysis of senescence, cellular senescence is a state that cells are compelled to enter due to external pressures like DNA damage, ectopic oncogene expression, and excessive cell proliferation to replace those lost to external/environmental factors.

Suppose there are enough of these senescent cells. In that case, they will likely result in tissue degeneration, which is thought to be an indication of organism aging. Senescence and aging, as determined by the epigenetic clock, are different processes at the cellular level. It is a built-in mechanism that has been in place since the beginning of the cell. This suggests that cells would still age even if the extrinsic pressures mentioned above do not cause them to enter senescence. This is in line with the findings that mice with naturally long telomeres nonetheless age and eventually die, despite having telomere lengths that are far longer than the critical limit, and that forcing telomere shortening causes replicative senescence, causes animals to age prematurely. As a result, cellular senescence is a process by which cells depart from aging naturally too soon.

Effects of race/ethnicity and gender

According to epigenetic age acceleration in the blood, brain, and saliva, males age more quickly than women, but it also depends on the lifestyle.

The epigenetic clock approach can be used to investigate all racial and ethnic groups because DNA age and chronological age are closely related. Ethnicity, however, may be linked to an epigenetic age acceleration. For instance, the Tsimané and Hispanic blood ages more slowly than the blood of other populations, which could account for the Hispanic mortality paradox.

Stem cell therapy's rejuvenating effects on the blood

The epigenetic age of blood is brought up to par with that of the donor through hematopoietic stem cell transplantation, which transfers these cells from a youthful donor to an older recipient. However, increasing DNA methylation age is linked to graft-versus-host disease.

Progeria

Epigenetic age acceleration is linked to adult progeria, also known as Werner syndrome, in blood. samples of fibroblasts taken from kids with Hutchinson-Gilford According to the "skin & blood" epigenetic clock, progeria demonstrate accelerated epigenetic aging effects, although not following the original pan tissue clock from Horvath.

The biological system underlying the epigenetic clock

The specific biological process underlying the epigenetic clock is currently unknown, even though biomarkers of aging based on DNA methylation data have enabled precise age estimations for any tissue over the entire life span.

However, epigenetic biomarkers may be able to answer several lingering issues, including the essential query of why we age. Therefore, it would be prudent to compare and determine the relationship between the readings of the epigenetic clock and the transcriptome aging clock to comprehend the fundamentals of the mechanisms underlying the epigenetic clock. The following justifications have now been offered in the literature.

1. Weidner et al. (2014) offer an age estimator for blood DNA utilizing only three CpG sites of genes that are hardly affected by aging (cg25809905 in integrin, alpha 2b (ITGA2B); cg02228185 in aspartoacylase (ASPA); and cg17861230 in phosphodiesterase 4C, cAMP-specific (PDE4C)). The gene integer has these three CpG sites.

Weidener et al. (2014).'s age estimator only works with blood. Applying this sparse estimator to data produced by the Illumina 27K or 450K platforms results in significantly less accurate results than Horvath's epigenetic clock (Horvath 2014), even in the blood. The sparse estimator, however, was created for pyrosequencing data and is quite economical.

2. Hannum et al. (2013) offer a different age estimation for each tissue type. Each of these estimators needs knowledge of the covariates (e.g., gender, body mass index, batch). The authors

note that every tissue produced a distinct linear offset (intercept and slope). As a result, the scientists used a linear model to modify the blood-based age estimator for each tissue type. Figure 4A in Hannum et al. shows that when the Hannum estimator is used on different tissues, it results in a significant error (caused by inadequate calibration) (2013). As a result, the researchers altered the blood-based age estimator for each kind of tissue using a linear model. Hannum et al's 4A demonstrates that the Hannum estimator produces a considerable inaccuracy when applied to various tissues (due to insufficient calibration) (2013). The epigenetic clock, in contrast, differs in that one does not need to perform such a calibration step because it consistently employs the same CpGs and coefficacy figures. In order to compare the ages of multiple tissues, cells, and organs from the same person, Horvath's epigenetic clock can be employed. The age estimators from Hannum et al. can be used to compare the ages of malignant tissues with those of matching normal (non-cancerous) tissues. Still, they cannot be used to compare the ages of various normal tissues. In all malignancies, Hannum et al. showed strong age acceleration effects. Horvath's epigenetic clock, on the other hand, according to, some cancer forms (such as triple-negative breast malignancies and uterine corpus endometrial carcinoma) show negative age acceleration, meaning that cancer tissue may be much younger than anticipated. Additional covariates are a significant difference. Hannum's age estimators use gender, body mass index, diabetes status, ethnicity, and batch factors. One cannot apply it immediately to new data because it involves separate batches of data. The authors do, however, include coefficient values for their CpGs in Supplementary Tables that can be used to build an aggregate measure that frequently has a poor calibration but is substantially connected with chronological age (i.e., lead to high errors).

3. Giuliani et al. pinpoint the genomic sites in human teeth where DNA methylation levels are correlated with age. They suggest examining the DNA methylation levels at the ELOVL2, FHL2, and PENK genes in DNA extracted from the pulp and cementum of identical modern teeth. [66]They intend to use this technique on historical and comparatively old human teeth.

4. Using more than 6,000 blood samples, Galkin et al. trained an epigenetic aging clock with exceptional accuracy using deep neural networks.

The clock forecasts that persons with particular illnesses, such as IBD, frontotemporal dementia, ovarian cancer, and obesity, will be older than healthy controls using data from 1000 CpG sites. The aging clock will be made available to the general public in 2021 by the Deep Longevity Corporation, an Insilico Medicine offshoot.

The most accurate methods for analyzing DNA methylation in the clinic were compared by 18 research groups from three continents as part of a multicenter benchmarking study, which concluded that epigenetic tests based on DNA methylation are a mature technology ready for widespread clinical use.

Plasminogen activator inhibitor 1 (PAI1), which has been demonstrated to have higher connections with cardiometabolic disease than some epigenetic clocks, can also be utilized as an age estimator about DNA methylation levels, according to McCartney et al.

De Lima Camillo and others (2022) A highly precise and reliable pan-tissue epigenetic clock was developed using an optimized deep neural network. To obtain one of the lowest reported median absolute errors for human epigenetic age prediction of 2.153 years, the predictor, termed AltumAge, was trained on 142 datasets and uses 20,318 CpG sites. Horvath's linear technique performed better because AltumAge can identify CpG-CpG connections. For those with autism, HIV, multiple sclerosis, non-alcoholic fatty liver disease, type 2 diabetes, and atherosclerosis, AltumAge predicts a later age. AltumAge forecasts that cancer will age more slowly than healthy tissues than Horvath's clock. The clock's source code is accessible to everyone.

Various species

If mice and people undergo similar patterns of change in the methylome with age, Wang et al. [in mice livers] and Petkovich et al. [based on mice blood DNA methylation profiles] investigated. They discovered that mice given lifespan-extension treatments (such as calorie restriction or dietary rapamycin) had epigenetic ages that were noticeably younger than those of their untreated, wild-type age-matched controls. Moreover, mice age predictors also detect the lifespan effects of gene knockouts and the rejuvenation of fibroblast-derived iPSCs.

The median absolute error for the mice multi-tissue age prediction based on DNA methylation at 329 distinct CpG sites was less than four weeks (or 5% of a lifetime). The human clock is not entirely conserved in mice, as evidenced by an attempt to forecast age using the human clock sites in mice. The fact that the clocks in humans and mice differ shows that different species require different training methods for epigenetic clocks.

The aging of wild European lobster populations (Homarus Gammarus) using a unique technique that relies on a ribosomal DNA methylation-based clock was described in 2021.

In both domestic and wild animals, changes in DNA methylation patterns hold great promise for age estimation and biomarker discovery.

Potential for diet and lifestyle changes to reverse the effects of epigenetic aging

Given the societal and healthcare expenditures associated with an aging population, efforts to decrease biological aging and increase health span are of interest. Here, we present the results of a clinical experiment involving 43 healthy adult males between 50 and 72. The 8-week treatment plan included advice on diet, sleep, exercise, and relaxation, as well as probiotic and phytonutrient supplements. The control group received no assistance. Saliva samples were subjected to genome-wide DNA methylation analysis using the Illumina Methylation Epic Array, and damage was determined using the online Horvath DNAmAge clock (2013). Compared to controls, the food and lifestyle intervention reduced DNAmAge by 3.23 years (p=0.018). By the end of the program, the DNAmAge of those in the treatment group had fallen by an average of

1.96 years compared to the same people at the beginning, with a clear trend towards significance (p=0.066). In addition, mean serum 5-methyltetrahydrofolate (+15 percent, p=0.004) and mean triglycerides (-25 percent, p=0.009) showed substantial changes in blood biomarkers, this is the first randomized controlled trial to demonstrate that certain dietary and lifestyle changes may help healthy adult males slow down their epigenetic aging, as Horvath DNAmAge (2013) suggested. These results must be confirmed by larger, longer-lasting clinical trials and research on other human populations.

Aging is the biggest risk factor for decreased physical and mental ability and numerous non- communicable diseases such as cancer, neurodegeneration, type 2 diabetes, and cardiovascular disease. Our increasingly aging population poses an increasing number of health-related economic and social difficulties that impact individuals, their families, health systems, and economies. Economics alone shows that postponing aging by 2.2 years (and the resulting increase in health span) might result in a $7 trillion savings over the next fifty years. This comprehensive strategy was a significantly better investment than investing in individual diseases. Therefore, there will be significant benefits for public health and healthcare costs if interventions that even slightly lengthen the health span can be found.

DNA methylation is known to add a methyl group to cytosine residues at specific locations on a chromosome (such as CpG islands, shelf/shore, exons, and open sea). Methylation is the most thoroughly explored mechanism influencing gene expression and perhaps most durable. DNA methylation is the only epigenetic marker that can be easily and affordably mapped from tissue samples. A few thousand of the 20+ million methylation sites in the human genome show a strong correlation between methylation levels and age. The best biochemical age indicators available now are all based on methylation patterns. This has prompted some researchers to hypothesize that aging results from methylation alterations and other epigenetic changes that occur over time.

The multi-tissue DNAmAge clock is the methylation-based clock that has received the most research as of this writing. There were few practical alternatives at the time this study design was approved. Chronological age does not perform as well as Horvath's DNAmAge clock in predicting all-cause mortality and other morbidities. clocks for methylation such as DNAmAge, are based on age-related, systematic methylation alterations. In particular, the DNAmAge clock shows that around 60% of CpG sites experience methylation loss with aging, and 40% experience methylation gain. This is different from stochastic alterations, such as "methylation drift," which are unpredictable changes that vary from person to person and cell to cell within a person. Hypermethylation in tumor suppressor gene promoter regions (which inhibits production) and hypomethylation (which promotes inflammatory cytokines) are examples of systemic methylation alterations (promoting expression). White blood and buccal cells can be found in saliva, a strong source of high-quality DNA and an appropriate tissue type to be evaluated by the DNAmAge clock.

Because few dietary connections with the DNAmAge clock have been demonstrated, the food recommendations used as part of the therapy regimen for this investigation were mostly based on biochemistry and broad indicators of health. Blood carotenoids have shown a slight but significant reduction in DNAmAge in people who follow general lean meat, fish, and a plant- based diet. However, it's likely that adjustments with a bigger impact call for a more focused strategy. Therefore, the dietary intervention used in this study was also plant-centered. Still, it also included a high intake of nutrients that are substrates or cofactors in methylation biosynthetic pathways (such as folate and betaine), as well as cofactors and modulators for the enzyme ten-eleven translocation (TET) demethylase (such as alpha-ketoglutarate, vitamin C, and vitamin A) and polyphenolic DNA methyl transferase (DNMT There were also a few animal proteins that were high in nutrients (e.g., liver, egg). To reduce glycemic cycling, the diet limited carbs and included brief periods of intermittent fasting. In addition, a probiotic containing 40 million CFU of Lactobacillus Plantarum 299v and a fruit and vegetable powder high in polyphenolic modulators of DNMT activity was added to the diet regularly. In the presence of para-aminobenzoic acid (PABA), L. Plantarum has been proven to generate folate, and it has also been shown to change gene expression.

At least 30 minutes of daily activity, five days a week at least, at a level of intensity between 60 and 80 percent of maximum perceived effort, was recommended as part of the study's lifestyle recommendations. Exercise has been found to increase mean lifespan in animal models and is well recognized to be generally helpful for every area of health. Exercise's impact on the methylome is currently being investigated. For instance, 500 women who practiced tai chi regularly saw a slowdown in age-related DNA methylation reductions. A lifelong history of the exercise was linked to a comparable endpoint in a different trial with 647 women. As the Horvath clock was not yet created, these results were not reported in terms of it. Regular daily exercise was linked to decrease blood levels of homocysteine, which when elevated indicates a deficiency in methylation ability, according to a systematic analysis of human research. Even though this risk has only been seen in elite, competitive athletes, excessive exercise may speed up methylation aging.

For stress reduction, twice-daily breathing techniques that trigger the Relaxation Response were recommended. The Zombie-Piekarska clock was used to assess DNAmAge, and it was recently shown that 60 days of relaxation practice meant to evoke the Relaxation Response, 20 minutes twice per day, may considerably lower DNAmAge in their group of healthy volunteers (but not in their 'sick' group). The fact that 85 out of 353 DNAmAge CpG sites are found in glucocorticoid response elements suggests that stress and accelerated aging are likely related. The methylome has been found to age more quickly throughout a lifetime of cumulative stress. Dexamethasone, a glucocorticoid agonist, has also been shown to speed up the DNAmAge clock and cause-related transcriptional alterations, according to Zannas et al. Dexamethasone-regulated genes revealed an enhanced connection with age-related illnesses, such as leukemias, arteriosclerosis, and coronary artery disease. Other data show that PTSD causes the methylation age to accelerate and that greater newborn distress (lack of caregiver contact) is linked to a younger, undeveloped epigenetic age.

The important of this study was to improve sleep, and it suggested getting at least seven hours per night. The recommended amount of sleep every night is seven hours, but the scant research on accelerated aging only looks at cases of extreme sleep deprivation. Lack of sleep has influenced blood's genome-wide methylation patterns (likely a temporary one). In a group of 2078 women, sleeplessness has been linked to an accelerated DNAmAge clock. In a small sample of 12 female college students, Carskadon et al. discovered a correlation between poor sleep quality, fewer hours of sleep, and age acceleration.

This multimodal ("systems") intervention reflects a clinically-applied strategy that combines discrete therapies, each of which has been shown to positively impact the DNA methylome and of which multiple authors of this work have had clinical success in improving health. Such actions are likely to have synergistic effects and lessen the chance that the bad impacts of one factor promoting disease would offset the positive effects of another promoting health. As applied here, dietary and lifestyle therapies concentrate on upstream factors typically regarded as secure over a long period.

Horvath's DNAmAge clock was intended to be a key goal of this study, to see if it could possibly be slowed. This means that we have hesitantly agreed with the theory of methylation.

We anticipate that trying to directly affect the DNA methylome via diet and lifestyle to set back DNAmAge will result in a healthier, more "youthful" metabolism because the pattern from which the DNAmAge clock is computed is a driver of aging (and the chronic diseases of aging). Three uncontrolled investigations have thus far shown a DNAmAge setback. One tiny pilot study employing growth hormone, metformin,

DHEA, and two nutritional supplements was claimed to have slowed the DNAmAge clock in healthy men over 12 months by 1.5 (plus the one year of the study). Two further studies have shown that food and/or dietary supplement interventions can reduce age. Following a year of a Mediterranean diet and 400 IU of vitamin D3, a subgroup of Polish women from the NU-AGE cohort suggested a reduction in biological age of 1.47 years, and a 16-week trial using 4000 IU of vitamin D3 in overweight or obese African Americans with suboptimal D status revealed a 1.85-year reduction in biological age.

Here, we present comparable preliminary findings from eight-week diet and lifestyle treatments (preceded by a one-week education period).

CHAPTER 18

CLOCK FOR DNA METHYLATION

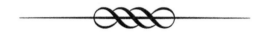

After the eight-week program, participants in the treatment group had an average Horvath DNAmAge clock score of 3.23 years younger than that of participants in the control group (n=20; p=0.018). At the end of the program, those in the treatment group (n=18) scored 1.96 years younger on average than those who did at the beginning, with a significant tendency

Towards significance (p=0.066 for within-group change). At the end of the study period, control participants scored on average 1.27 years older, although this within-group increase was not statistically significant (p= 0.153). DNAmAge change comparison between treatment and control groups

One of the characteristics of mammalian aging, from the loss of particular cell types to the diminished capacity for tissue repair, is a lowered stem cell function. It is simple to understand how methylation drift, which limits the adaptability of aging stem cells, can contribute to deteriorating tissue health. The onset of autoimmune illnesses is another hallmark of aging, and as was previously said, it's likely that age-related methylation drift contributes to this phenomenon by exposing tissue antigens that have been secreted or by changing lymphocyte function through hypomethylation. Other scenarios, such as the production of local inflammation or fibrosis, are also conceivable in which changes in a small number of cells could lead to considerable disease. Thus, epigenetic factors may play a role in a number of age- related diseases.

The abnormal focused stem cell proliferation that results from epigenetic variation at the tissue level may be one of its most significant impacts. Cancer and atherosclerotic heart disease, the two leading causes of death in people, are both focused proliferative processes. Focal proliferation itself causes disease, as in coronary atherosclerosis, in tissues with relatively low cellular turnover, low levels of carcinogen exposure, and few spontaneous mutations. It's interesting to note that atherosclerotic plaques have abnormal methylation of genes like ERa and ERb. The age-related clonal expansion may enable oncogenic mutations to change cells, leading to full-blown malignancy, in tissues that are frequently exposed to carcinogens, such as the lung or gastrointestinal tract. The convergence of age-related epigenetic drift and carcinogen-induced genetic change may be the primary explanation for the rise in the incidence of cancer as people age, keeping in mind that the majority of oncogenic mutations (such as the activating KRAS mutation) result in senescence or death of normal cells. Indeed, genome-wide investigations have now demonstrated that concurrent genetic and epigenetic damage is a feature of malignancies.

Cancer offers a vivid illustration of how aging, epigenetic drift, and disease interact. Numerous epigenetic changes, including abnormal DNA methylation, are seen in cancer cells. Studying normal-appearing tissues close to cancer allowed researchers to identify increased promoter CpG island methylation in aging normal cells, which was then proposed to be an early stage of carcinogenesis. If stem cell replication is viewed as the pinnacle of the biologic clock, then.

154

Approximately 70–80 percent of the DNA methylation anomalies in cancer can be linked to aging faults. Cancer itself can also be viewed as an accelerated aging event. These descriptive investigations are supported by direct, compelling evidence that links epigenetic errors to oncogenesis. First, there is an inverse correlation between genetic and epigenetic defects at these loci, suggesting an equivalent growth advantage regardless of the molecular defect.

Second, some of the genes altered epigenetically in cancer are genuine tumor suppressor genes that result in familial cancer clusters when mutated. Second, the epigenetic code's authors, editors, and readers are frequently altered in cancer, indicating that the neoplastic phenotype is functionally caused by downstream epigenetic abnormalities. Last but not least, in mice models, increasing methylation by overexpressing Dnmt3b reduces polyp formation while decreasing methylation in the normal colon is achieved by partial deletion of Dnmt1. These findings are consistent with the model's assertion that some preneoplastic lesions develop at a rate limited by age-related methylation abnormalities. Cancers are frequently reported to develop in areas of aberrant DNA methylation in human carcinogenesis, which is also compatible with the hypothesis.

Metabolic assessments

Over the eight-week research period, the mean triglycerides decreased by 25%, from 112 to 89 mg/dL (p=0.009), which was the most significant improvement in blood indicators. In addition, the mean serum 5-methyltetrahydrofolate (5-MTHF) increased 15% from 78 to 88 nmol/L (p=0.004), as anticipated from a diet high in folate.

None of the other blood markers assessed (glucose, hemoglobin A1C, total cholesterol, HDL cholesterol, LDL cholesterol, methionine, s-adenosylmethionine (SAM), s- adenosylhomocysteine (SAH), the ratio SAM: SAH, and homocysteine) changed significantly compared to controls, but within-group analysis revealed a significant decrease in total cholesterol (-22.8 mg/d

Emotional controls

The PROMIS indices of emotional wellbeing between the treatment and control groups did not differ statistically after controlling for baseline values. There was a trend toward lower anxiety scores in the therapy group, but these changes were not statistically significant.

These results are significant for many reasons, but notably, they represent the first instance of possible epigenetic age reversal in a randomized, controlled clinical experiment that took into account any typical variation in epigenetic methylation. This is the second account of how a change in food and lifestyle slows biological aging in people otherwise known to be healthy.

The fact that this study was conducted over a shorter period and that the scale of possible Decrease was modest but may have considerable socioeconomic advantages to society is noteworthy.

In overweight/obese African Americans with a blood 25-hydroxyvitamin D [25(OH)d] level of 50 nmol/L, vitamin D3 at a dose of 4,000 IU/d for 16 weeks has been demonstrated to reduce DNAmAge clock measurement by 1.85 years [31]. The DNAmAge clock was then demonstrated to be advanced by 1.5 years in 9 middle-aged males following a one-year program of daily growth hormone injections with one prescription medication and three nutritional supplements (plus the one-year study length = 2.5 years) [29]. More recently, a 1-year non-controlled pilot trial involving 120 participants aged 65 to 79 from the larger NU-AGE cohort (including 60 Italians and 60 Poles) revealed a non-significant trend toward DNAmAge clock reversal following the consumption of 400 IU of vitamin D3 along with a Mediterranean diet. Subgroup analysis did, however, show a significant 1.47-year age drop among Polish female participants (n=36) and in people with a higher epigenetic age at baseline. Poland is a nation with a non- Mediterranean baseline diet, the study revealed. Using similarly non-invasive and usually helpful therapies known to have molecular plausibility for changing methylation pathways, biological age setback was achieved in the current study in eight weeks.

The rise in circulation folate shows that food sources and probiotics that produce folate are viable options for nutritional replacement. With a diet that reduces carbohydrate intake, glycemic response, and exercise, a decrease in blood triglycerides may be anticipated. The average starting homocysteine value of the treatment group was 10.9 umol/L, already within the range that is typically considered to be "normal" (15 umol/L), even though we expected to see a decrease in homocysteine with an intervention that provided additional dietary B vitamins and betaine, as well as exercise.

DNA methylation's effects on non-methyl donor factors

We came to learn that nutrition factors might modify DNA methylation marks in such a way as to suppress gene expression and significantly alter phenotype through the pioneering work of Waterland and Jirtle in the Agouti mouse model. Over the ensuing years, the ability of nutrition to affect revolutionary phenotypic changes has persisted, most significantly in animal research and a few small human trials. All of the aforementioned human trials (NU-AGE, TRIIM, Vitamin D3 study, etc.) and the current study were able to alter DNA methylomes without the use of extra-dietary supplements of well-known methyl donor foods (such as folate, vitamin B12, choline, SAMe, or betaine), supporting the idea of a broad regulatory network on DNA methylation and marking a change from earlier studies that more directly altered DNA methylation with the use of extra-

A net increase in methylation is not the treatment objective, as opposed to changing methylation at the proper sties, because the DNAmAge clock is calculated from some sites that increase and others that decrease methylation with age. The recommended diet included TET demethylase-associated nutrients, such as vitamins A and C, and particular plant polyphenols, such as curcumin and EGCG, known to inhibit DNMT activity, in addition to high levels of food- sourced methyl donor nutrients because this study focused on a healthy methylation pattern rather than just increased methylation. Younger DNAmAge (i.e., "improved" methylation patterns) in the treatment group without a general increase (or decrease) in methylation suggests that these compounds work together to boost methylation and demethylation enzyme support and, as a result, may be able to control where methyl groups are applied and removed. Additionally, it has been demonstrated that combining polyphenols rather than using a single phytonutrient has enhanced positive effects on epigenetic alterations.

Reasons against supplementing with methyl donor nutrients

The current study's design carefully avoided extra-dietary supplementation of nutrients that act as methyl donors because a growing body of epidemiological data suggests potential long-term hazards, to which the short-term studies were not sensitive. Multiple trials have discovered a positive association between methyl donor supplementation and increased cancer risk, even though overall data are conflicting and some conditions (such as pregnancy, macrocytic anemia, hyperhomocysteinemia, and dietary restrictions) frequently necessitate extra-dietary supplementation: A published long-term follow-up on 2,524 participants in the B-PROOF trial found an increased risk of colorectal cancer in particular (HR 1.77, 95 percent CI 1.08-2.90, p=0.02) and overall cancer (HR 1.25, 95 percent CI 1.00-1.53) after 2-3 years of daily supplementation with 400 mcg folic acid and 500 mcg vitamin B12. According to a meta- analysis of 2 trials conducted in Norway, taking 400 mg of vitamin B12 daily in addition to 800 mcg of folic acid was linked to a higher risk of death from any cause and cancer. Contrarily, baseline dietary folate intake was found to be inversely associated with prostate cancer risk in a trial that later revealed an increased risk of prostate cancer in the treatment arm that received 1 mg of folic acid per day for 10 years, and baseline dietary folate intake was discovered to be negatively correlated with the development of non-muscle-invasive bladder cancer in a study that also discovered increased recurrence for folic acid consumption. A vitamin D and calcium intervention with the addition of folic acid, vitamin B6, and vitamin B12 dietary supplements sped up biological aging (sex-adjusted odds ratio 5.26 vs. However, this was only seen in small research.

Precautions and next steps

The comparatively small sample size of this pilot study has a substantial impact on its statistical power. It is, therefore, necessary to confirm these findings in larger research populations and populations other than middle-aged males.

It is yet unclear whether treatments that slow one or more of the "methylation clocks" inherently reduce the likelihood of developing age-related diseases. Epidemiologists continue to focus on this question as they attempt to validate the predictors of age-related morbidity and mortality, which would otherwise require extremely lengthy clinical trials. As was already mentioned, there are benefits to using a multimodal strategy, but it also implies that it is impossible to credit better results to any particular aspect of the intervention. The combination of interventions utilized in this study could be strengthened and made to have a greater impact by adding additional personalization. Future revisions of the intervention will focus on improving the program's effectiveness, efficiency, scalability, and affordability in ongoing clinical trials. Such food and lifestyle therapies will probably undergo adjustments as our knowledge of the individualized application of these interventions grows, which may further extend biological aging markers.

Finally, new "omics" methods may help us comprehend biological age prediction and reversal in ways other than DNA methylation alone. Therefore, it is important to consider integrating

multi-omics data in future studies of potential age-delaying therapies.

Between March 2018 and August 2019, 43 adult males between 50 and 72 eligible and with no recent or chronic medical history were recruited, given their consent, enrolled, and randomly assigned. Figure 3 displays a CONSORT flowchart. To eliminate the potential confounding effect of pre-, peri-and post-menopausal sex hormone levels of the same age range in women, the age range of 50–72 was chosen as the time when age-related vulnerabilities often show.

All participants had a 3-week washout period (with written instructions) during which they were instructed to stop using any dietary supplements or herbal remedies that had not been recommended by a qualified healthcare professional for a medical problem. Low dose supplements, like the typical "1-a-day" multivitamin/mineral (high potency, high dose multivitamin/mineral products were not allowed), and/or other supplements taken for prevention, like fish oil (up to 1 gram/day), vitamin D (up to 6000 IU/day), vitamin C (up to 1g/day), and vitamin E (up to 400 IU/day), were acceptable exceptions for dietary supplementation. Even though these supplements were neither advised nor prescribed, participants were permitted to continue using them throughout the study to record any

impacts on their baseline ratings. In addition, the participants consented to abstain from or stop using any recreational drugs or substances, as well as to refrain from using alcohol, nicotine, marijuana, or cannabinoids at least one week before the start of the study.

At the baseline visit, study participants were randomly assigned using a specific randomization sequence (randomization.com). Opening sealed, signed envelopes created by research workers unrelated to the study that were only opened at randomization allowed for the concealment of allocations.

At visit 1, basic training and recorded webinars on technology and instruction were given. Participants in the treatment group were told to start the 8-week intervention plan, which includes dietary, supplement, and lifestyle adjustments, one week following the baseline visit to give time for participant education. At each of the three study visits, saliva samples were taken (baseline, week 5, and week 9).

At visits 1 and 2, Metagenics Inc., 25 Enterprise Aliso Viejo, CA 92656 USA, provided two dietary supplements (PhytoGanix and UltraFlora Intensive Care). At visits 2 and 3, unused medications were gathered, tallied, and recorded. In addition, dosage compliance was examined retrospectively using returned doses, directly questioned about each interventional element during study visits, and frequently in touch with trial participants.

Regular coaching sessions were provided to encourage program adherence, administered weekly for the first four weeks and at least every other week after that. Coaching sessions adhered to a predetermined script that covered medication modifications and adherence to intervention standards. In addition, MBody360, 640 Broadway 5A, New York, NY 10012, offered a HIPAA-compliant electronic technology coaching tool that included reference guidelines, menu planning suggestions, optional recipes, and a shopping list. This feature allowed participants to contact their assigned coach between planned coaching sessions. Participants who were unable or unable to use MBody360 had additional options, including email, web platforms, and/or phone communication

CHAPTER 19

CALCULATING EPIGENETIC AGE

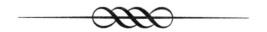

Saliva samples were handled carefully and kept frozen at -70° C for the length of the trial. After clinical operations, frozen samples were batch sent overnight on dry ice to Yale University Center for Genome Analysis. Sample IDs were assigned to plates before shipment to equally distribute measurement-related random variability across plates. Hence, each plate contained a representative assortment of samples from both allocation groups (treatment and control) and a distribution of samples from each trial visit.

Extraction of DNA

DNA was extracted from Oragene Saliva tubes using the Perkin Elmer Chemagic 360 Instrument (kit# CMG-1081) following the manufacturer's suggested procedure. Following the 50-degree Celsius Oragene Saliva Incubation, 80 mL of 4 mg/g American Bioanalytical RNASE A (Part#AB12023-00100) was applied before loading samples into the equipment.

Genome-wide RNA and DNA

A260/A280 and A260/A230 ratios (provided by the Nanodrop 1000 Spectrophotometer), both of which should be > 1.8, were used to assess the RNA/purity. DNA's the gel electrophoresis pattern matched up with samples that didn't deteriorate.

Methods

Sample DNA was standardized to the Zymo EZ-96 DNA Methylation Kit's suggested starting concentration of 1 g. (Cat No D5004). The materials were purified using the Zymo Methylation procedure after being converted to bisulfate overnight. The Illumina Infinium HD assay (Illumina Methylation Epic Array Cat. No. WG-317-1001) was used to amplify the whole genome overnight at 37 degrees Celsius on the samples. The next day, samples were fragmented for an hour at 37 degrees, precipitated for 30 minutes at 4 degrees, and pelleted for 20 minutes at 3000xg at 4 degrees. Following Illumina's Infinium HD assay at 48 degrees Celsius, samples were re-suspended in the necessary volume of RA1 and dried in a hood for 1 hour at room temperature. The samples were then denatured for 20 minutes at 95 degrees Celsius. Finally, samples were directly hybridized to the Illumina Methylation Epic Array Cat. No. WG-317-1001 after a 10-minute cooling period. Each chip's sample placement was random. A stable hybridization oven was used for the 18-hour process, which was carried out at 48 degrees Celsius. The Tecan Freedom Evo technology automatically washed and stained the arrays the next day. The UV shield (Illumina's XC3) was applied to the arrays for 10 minutes, and any excess was wiped off. Arrays were vacuum desiccated for an hour to dry them out. The Scan array scanner from Illumina was used to scan the arrays, producing raw files. Illumina's Genome Studio software was used to import raw data files, construct a project, and check the QC settings to ensure everything went as planned. Using Illumina's Genome Studio, scanned output files were examined, and call rates were calculated. Both samples dependent and sample independent controls assessed the data's quality. The effectiveness of target removal, non- specific binding, and cross-contamination appearance was specifically studied. The password-protected Keck Microarray Database was used to upload the Genome Studio project and its raw Data.

Data analysis

The online Horvath clock at https://dnamage.genetics.ucla.edu/ was used to determine DNAmAge. The remaining 18 people in the treatment group and 20 participants in the control group were subjected to a blinded analysis of epigenetic age. Individual score differences (after treatment minus before) were used as a random variable to calculate the individual t-test P values between the experimental and control groups.

Epigenetic Reprogramming Can Turn Back the Clock on Aging

Birthday candles are not a reliable indicator of either human health or longevity, as aging specialists are aware. However, the genome contains a wealth of information, and animal experiments have shown that some age-related damage can be reversed by eliminating or reprogramming troublesome cells or inhibiting the action of viral proteins.

As it turns out, DNA methylation, a frequently used indicator of biological age, "really controls time within cells" rather than just noting time like a clock on the wall, says David Sinclair, a Harvard Medical School aging researcher and cofounder of 4-year-old Life Biosciences.

The finding was made as a consequence of a recent study from Harvard scientists that were published in Nature (DOI: 10.1038/s41586-020-2975-4). In this work, the Harvard researchers showed for the first time that the pattern of DNA methylation in the genome may be safely reset to a younger age.

Sinclair, who has devoted most of his adult life to researching the epigenetic alterations brought on by aging, claims that it was, in fact, a requirement for restoring youthful function and vision in old mice. He believed the process was unidirectional and that cells eventually lost their identity, malfunctioned, or developed cancer until a few years ago.

According to Sinclair, trying to persuade proteins to return to where they were in developing cells "seemed ridiculous." Scientists were unsure whether proteins could be reversed, where the instructions were stored, or whether they were being stored. Proteins move about in response to age-associated DNA damage and end up in the incorrect locations on the genome, leading the incorrect genes to be turned on.

Sinclair now thinks that aging is caused by epigenetic alterations confusing the body's ability to interpret genetic code, as detailed in his 2019 best-seller Lifespan. He compares the procedure to retrieving music from a scratched CD and adds that they are essentially searching for the polish to enable the cell to read the DNA correctly once more.

CHAPTER 20

YAMANAKA ELEMENTS

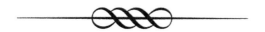

Because retinal tissues begin deteriorating soon after birth, Sinclair and his research colleagues have been concentrating on the eye. An injured optic nerve can recover in a baby, but the damage is permanent at age one.

He continues that Yuncheng Lu, a former student of Sinclair's, was particularly intrigued by the eye because his family has a business that corrects vision, and he saw blindness as a "major unmet need." "We thought we may be able to witness regrowth of the optic nerve if it was destroyed if we could take the age of those retinal cells back far enough, but not so far that they lose their identity."

A 2016 study in Cell (DOI: 10.1016/j.cell.2016.11.052) by Life Biosciences cofounder Juan Carlos Izpisua Belmonte (Salk Institute for Biological Studies) turned on "Yamanaka factors" Oct4, Sox2, Klf4, and c-Myc (OSKM) highly expressed in embryonic stem cells partially erased cellular markers of aging in mice that aged prematurely as well as in human cells. Moreover, in the short-lived mice, short-term induction of OSKM reduced signs of aging and somewhat increased lifespan.

Since the mice perished if the therapy lasted longer than two days, Sinclair claims that the lifetime increase was commonly regarded as "an artifact of shocking a mouse." Nevertheless, his Harvard team chose to test the strategy by utilizing an adeno-associated virus as a vehicle to transfer the youth-restoring OSKM genes into the retinas of aging mice, even if the effects on human health seemed implausible.

It wasn't until Lu decided to remove the c-Myc gene, an oncogene, from his research using human skin cells that the technique stopped killing the mice or making them develop cancer. He observed [damaged] cells that had been producing OSK for three weeks and noticed an incredible amount of nerve growth back toward the brain. Furthermore, the treatment made the cells younger while the harm made them older.

The trio of Yamanaka factors effectively made cells younger without causing them to lose their identity (i.e., turn back into induced pluripotent stem cells) or promoting tumor growth even after a year of continuous treatment of a mouse's entire body, as the larger team went on to demonstrate in the Nature paper. Moreover, according to Sinclair, the mice had fewer tumors during the experiment.

Sinclair said the study will be repeated to determine whether the epigenetic reprogramming method can lengthen lifespan, even though the mice had to be autopsied to accurately estimate tumor burden.

According to Sinclair, the findings have ramifications beyond treating age-related eye illnesses. Researchers on aging have written studies demonstrating the ability to rejuvenate various tissues, such as kidney and muscle cells.

CHAPTER 21

CLOCKED OUTPUT

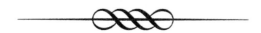

In the most recent mouse study, epigenetic reprogramming was discovered to have three advantageous impacts on the eye: promoting optic nerve regeneration, reversing vision loss in aging animals without glaucoma, and reversing vision loss with a disease matching human glaucoma. According to Sinclair, the latter result is the more significant. Ultimately, this is a tale about discovering a storehouse of youth-preserving knowledge within aging cells.

According to Sinclair, the findings of all three trials are remarkable and are "generally regarded to be three different processes." That is just a result of the fact that acute and chronic diseases and aging are separate disciplines with little interaction.

By tackling the fundamental cause, the Harvard team is developing a novel approach to treating aging-related disorders. According to Sinclair, this is the first instance where old animals were used to study nerve injury rather than young ones. Even though glaucoma is a disease of aging, age is often ignored in the cases of glaucoma and most disorders.

Because they are thought to be the most accurate predictors of biological age and future health, a variety of aging clocks, including several the study team constructed themselves, have been used for studies, adds Sinclair. In addition, for cells to remember their function throughout the next 80 to 100 years, they lay down various methylation patterns as embryos.

According to Sinclair, methyl groups reliably accumulate and withdraw from DNA bases in various cell and tissue types and even species for unidentified causes. According to how far above or below the DNA methylation line an individual sits, UCLA's Steve Horvath (another co- founder of Life Biosciences) demonstrated in 2013 that machine learning could be used to identify the "hot spots" and predict an individual's lifespan (Genome Biology, DOI: 10.1186/Gb- 2013-14-10-r115).

Since then, many different aging clocks have been created. Aging According to Sinclair, aging clocks are not particularly mysterious, but standards in the sector will eventually be necessary. ",

Increasing Field

Epigenetic reprogramming is expected to become a particularly busy area of Research on the rapidly expanding subject of aging. According to Sinclair, "there are still just a dozen or so labs working on this intensely, but perhaps a hundred others are getting into it."

He notes that while Life Biosciences initially had four labs, the number of new ones joining has increased virtually weekly. In addition to the eye, collaborators have extended their work to include the ear and more body parts.

He continues, "We're also orders of magnitude lowering the cost of the DNA clock test so [biological age prediction] can be done on millions of people. As a result, aging clocks are anticipated to become a common test in doctors' toolkits to direct patient care and track cancer treatment responses.

According to Sinclair, Life Biosciences has already received a license from Harvard University for two patents on the technologies employed by older researchers. In addition, the business has assembled a scientific team with a group of top-notch advisors who created gene therapy for the eye, which will be used to treat glaucoma as a starting point.

Recent Research revealed at a symposium that mice's lifespans can be significantly increased by fasting-induced autophagy, the cell's natural method for removing extra or malfunctioning components. She thinks that by initiating this process, disorders like macular degeneration and Alzheimer's may one day be treated.

CHAPTER 22

REVERSAL OF

HUMAN AGING TENDENCIES

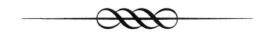

I n affluent nations, population aging is becoming a bigger problem associated with several medical, social, economic, political, and psychological issues. Many biological strategies to slow down aging have been studied in animal models over the past few years, and some of these appear to be able to reverse broad aging elements in adult animals based on a range of physiological parameters. Determinations of epigenetic age, which can offer a straightforward but persuasive indicator of biological as opposed to chronological age, can now provide a simple but compelling indication of age but have not yet supported any evidence that systemic aging can be reversed. Furthermore, it's important to address immunosenescence brought on by thymic involution. Thymic involution is associated with age-related increases in the incidence of cancer, infectious disease, autoimmune conditions, and generalized inflammation. It also results in the depletion of critical immune cell populations. On the other hand, centenarians exhibit preserved immunological activity. The total number of lymphoid precursors does not change with aging, but the migration of T-cell precursors from the bone marrow also seems to be dependent on thymic function, which is also dependent on the supply of T-cell progenitors from the bone marrow in aging.

For these reasons, in 2015–2017, we carried out the TRIIM (Thymus Regeneration, Immunorestoration, and Insulin Mitigation) trial, which may be the first human clinical trial to reverse components of human aging. The TRIIM trial's goal was to determine whether recombinant human growth hormone (rhGH) could be used to prevent or reverse immunosenescence in a group of men between the ages of 51 and 65 deemed healthy. This age range corresponds to the period just before the TCR repertoire begins to decline. Based on earlier Research showing that growth hormone (GH) had immune reconstituting and thixotropic effects in animals and human HIV patients, rhGH was employed. We coupled rhGH with dehydroepiandrosterone (DHEA) and metformin to reduce the "diabetogenic" effect of GH because GH-induced hyperinsulinemia is undesirable and might compromise thymic regeneration and immunological reconstitution. DHEA has numerous benefits that counteract the negative effects of natural aging in both men and women. Since metformin is a powerful calorie restriction mimic in old rats, it has been proposed as a potential treatment for slowing down human aging. However, it is unknown if DHEA or metformin alone can have any thixotropic effects.

RESULTS 2

Treatment side effects and safety

This study's main issue was if elevated IGF-1 levels could worsen malignant or precancerous foci in the prostate. PSA or percent-free PSA levels can be used to measure both of these changes. The overall index of prostate cancer risk, PSA, percent free PSA, and the ratio of PSA to percent free PSA did, however, significantly improve by day 15 of

173

treatment and remained favorably altered through the end of 12 months. After consulting the volunteers, a brief increase in PSA in two volunteers at 6 months was swiftly corrected and was understood to indicate recent sexual activity. Testosterone levels were unchanged.

Another major worry was that boosting immune activity might worsen age-related inflammation. However, therapy reduced CRP, and the decrease became statistically significant after 9 to 12 months. IL-6, a cytokine that promotes inflammation, did not change.

There were no significant changes in the serum levels of albumin, lipids, hematocrit, hemoglobin, platelet count, electrolytes, or liver enzymes. DHEA and metformin co-administration typically provided adequate control of insulin levels (although one outlier resulted in a rise in mean insulin at 12 months), and glucose levels remained stable. Finally, after 9–12 months (with a trend toward improvement at 18 months as well), estimated glomerular filtration rates (eGFR), which are important for the possibility of lactic acidosis with metformin as well as treatment success, showed a statistically significant improvement (Figure 1i). Except for two instances, side effects were minimal and typical with the administration of rhGH. There were two cases of arthralgias, one of anxiety, one of carpal tunnel syndrome, one of fluid retention, one of minor gynecomastia, and one of each of muscular soreness (1 case). Due to self-reported bradycardia before the trial and the delayed disclosure of a strong familial history of malignancy, one trial volunteer was removed from the study after around one month.

Regenerative responses in the bone marrow and the thymus

Figure 2 shows that the thymic MRI density has seen clear qualitative improvements. Based on the linear mixed-model analysis, the overall rise in the fat-free thymic fraction (TFFF) was quantifiably significant at the p = 8.57 1017 level, suggesting a recovery of thymic functional mass. In 7 out of 9 individuals, the changes were noticeable. The TFFFs of two participants did not substantially change after treatment (highest relative changes of +9.6 percent (p >.3) and

+12.4 percent (p >.2); Figure 3b), even though they had exceptionally low amounts of thymic fat (high TFFF) at baseline. In addition, they didn't respond, regardless of their age. Instead, regardless of baseline age, improvement in TFFF was dependent upon baseline TFFF.

Sternal BMFFF, on the other hand, grew significantly more slowly but consistently (Figure 3d; p

.001 for single-point comparison, or p = 9.5 1012 for formal linear mixed-model analysis), reaching high statistical significance. Like the thymus, bone marrow had a pattern of increasing BMFFF with higher baseline fat content, but the pattern's specifics differed (Figure 3f). This distinction, along with the stronger replacement of thymic fat compared to bone marrow fat, is consistent with both a specific reversal of thymic involution rather than a more generalized regression of body fat caused by GH administration and potential stimulation of bone marrow T-cell progenitor production.

Alterations in cytokines and immune cell subsets

The most significant alterations, according to an analysis of immune cell populations characterized by CyTOF, were found to be reductions in total and CD38-positive monocytes (Figure 4a, b), which led to an increase in the lymphocyte-to-monocyte ratio (LMR) (Figure 4c). After 9 and 12 months of treatment, a significant association was also found between TFFF and the decline in the percentage of CD38+ monocytes ($r2 =.59$, $p =.01$), as well as between TFFF and the ratio of lymphocytes to CD38+ monocytes ($r2 =.55$, $p =.018$). When correlated across all treatment durations, similar patterns were observed for total monocytes vs. TFFF and for the overall LMR vs. TFFF (respectively, $r2 =.40$, $p =.039$ and $r2 =.45$, $p =.019$). (0, 9, and 12 months). The increase in LMR was still highly significant at 18 months, and the alterations in mean monocyte populations lasted 6 months after treatment stopped ($p =.012$ for normalized CD38+ monocytes and $p =.022$ for normalized total monocytes).

With therapy, PD-1-positive CD8 T cells drastically decreased (Figure 4d). We were able to identify significant increases in both naive CD4 and naive CD8 T cells by gating on naive T cells (Figure 4e-f), as well as a significant ($p =.017$) rise in the proportion of CD31+CD45RA+CD4 T cells. + cells (CD4 RTEs, or recent thymic emigrants) during the therapy (linear correlation, Figure S1). We found no consistent alterations when senescent T cells were assessed as CD57+ or CD28-cells. However, a considerable rise in serum FGF-21 levels was found.

Epigenetic regression with age

According to the findings of all four epigenetic clocks (Figure 5a-d), epigenetic age was significantly reduced by treatment even though trial volunteers' epigenetic ages (EAs) were, on average, lower than their chronological ages (As) at baseline [(EA-A)0 0, Table 1], with a mean change in EA-A after 12 months of roughly 2.5 years (Figure 5e). Age at treatment initiation or (EA-A)0 had no impact on the treatment's effect on epigenetic age regression at 12 months (Table 1). For each clock, the linear mixed-model analysis (LMMA) results showed significant levels ranging from $p =.0009-.012$ for the months 0–12 to $p =.0016-.028$ for the months 0–18. (Figure 5 legend). After accounting for changes in blood cell composition, the Horvath clock LMMA results remained unchanged (p =.018). ((lymphocyte count, LMR, and the percentage of CD8 T cells that are senescent). At trial month 18, the average improvement was more than 1.5 years. Even though there was a general tendency for EA-A to trend back toward (EA-A)0 6 months following treatment withdrawal (Figure 5e, p.001). Additionally, the GrimAge clock, which can accurately forecast a person's life expectancy (Lu et al., 2019), showed no regression of (EA-A)-(EA-A)0 after therapy and a gain of almost 2.1 years at trial month 18 with 12 months still left (Figure 5d; Table 1). Additionally, a comparison of the rates of aging regression between 0-9 and 9-12 months revealed that, for every age estimator, the rate of aging regression appeared to significantly increase with lengthening treatment time (Figure 5a–d and Table 1), with a mean slope over all four clocks ranging from 1.56 0.46 years/year in the first 9 months to 6.48 0.34 years/year in the final 3 months of treatment (p .005, Figure 5f

DISCUSSION 3

The TRIIM study was created to reduce risks and adverse effects while examining the potential for thymus regeneration and reversing immunosenescent trends in healthy males. Our findings confirm the viability of this objective but unanticipatedly also provide compelling evidence that human beings can reverse several aging-related factors and biomarkers. These two findings might be connected.

Growth hormone therapy has been shown to reverse age-related immunological deficiencies and promote thymus regeneration and reactivation in aging rats and dogs by restoring youthful thymic histology (Goff, Roth, Arp, et al., 1987; Kelley et al., 1986). (Kelley et al., 1986). However, it has been questioned if human thymic tissue survives past the age of roughly 54, which is necessary for efficient thymus regeneration in elderly people (Simanovsky, Hiller, Loubashevsky, & Rozovsky, 2012). There is no information on whether regeneration was seen in people over 50 in the findings that show enhanced thymic CT density and immunological benefits brought on by rhGH in HIV patients, whose thymi are physiologically atypical (McCune et al., 1998). The current study now provides highly significant evidence of thymic regeneration in healthy aging men, along with improvements in several disease risk factors and age-related immunological parameters, as well as significant correlations between TFFF and positive changes in monocyte percentages and the LMR, independent of age up to 65 at the start of treatment. These findings align with the growth hormone's well-documented capacity to promote thymic epithelial cell proliferation and hematopoiesis (Savino, 2007). We feel this is a novel finding because our observation of an increase in FGF-21 levels after 12 months of treatment shows that the current treatment may be partially responsible for the thymic regeneration (Youm, Horvath, Mangelsdorf, Kliewer, & Dixit, 2016).

While DHEA treatment may actually raise monocyte levels, there is no evidence from prior studies linking rhGH administration to higher LMR or lower levels of monocytes (Khorram, Vu, & Yen, 1997). Although the underlying mechanisms are unclear, the unanticipated impact of our medication on the LMR may be extremely important for two reasons.

First, higher LMRs are linked to both better prognoses for a number of the leading causes of human mortality, such as at least 8 types of cancer [for example, prostate cancer; Caglayan et al., 2019], atherosclerosis; cardiovascular disease; and stroke; and are also linked to lower levels of overall inflammation. An LMR above 5 has been linked to protection from cardiovascular disease. Mean volunteer LMRs in our study were much higher at the end of treatment and six months after it than at baseline, when they were significantly lower.

The majority of monocytes are CD38-positive, which is the second factor. Age-related tissue NAD+ depletion appears to be primarily caused by increasing CD38 expression in mice and, most likely, in humans. CD38 is a NADase enzyme degrading the NAD+ precursor, nicotinamide mononucleotide. According to a recent study (Camacho-Pereira et al., 2016), age-related inflammation is thought to be the primary factor for the induction of CD38, which might theoretically include monocytes. No other CD38+ immune cell population was shown to have decreased in response to thymus regeneration treatment, even though many other immune cells express CD38, suggesting that monocytes may be particularly important. Therefore, the probability of a rise in tissue NAD+ levels is raised by our observation of a decrease in CRP combined with a decrease in monocyte levels. The exact mechanism by which CRP was decreased is unknown, but in theory, autoimmune-related inflammation may be lowered by reactivating negative selection in the thymus and clearing out pro-inflammatory viruses or senescent somatic cells. Given the link between age-related tissue NAD+ depletion and the development of aging phenotypes, our observations of reversed epigenetic aging, the general association of higher LMRs with better health, and prior findings linking thymus transplantation to regression of various nonimmunological aging processes could all be explained by an increase in tissue NAD+ content. Strong decreases in total and CD38+ monocytes, increases in LMR, and decreases in Grim Age were all seen to last for six months after treatment was stopped, which is consistent with this theory.

The possibility that thymus regeneration therapy epigenetically reprograms "exhausted" CD8 T cells (TEX), a recently identified unique PD-1+ CD8 population, is consistent with treatment- induced reductions in PD-1+ CD8 T cells. Due partly to PD-1, an immune checkpoint molecule that inhibits T-cell proliferative responses and is involved in cancer evasion of immune control, these cells are of great interest. Therefore, much effort is being put into creating pharmaceutical immune checkpoint inhibitors that specifically target PD-1. In addition, blocking PD-1 signaling improves the proliferation of "senescent" human CD-8 cells (Henson, Macaulay, Riddell, Nunn, & Akbar, 2015). Additionally, mice exhibit a PD-1+ and Tim-3+ subpopulation of worn-out CD8 cells that are associated with aging. Therefore, a decline in PD-1+ CD8 T cells after thymus regeneration therapy is probably indicative of a significant improvement in the immunological condition.

Our volunteer cohort was pre-immunosenescent and did not have baseline depletions of naive CD4 and CD8 T cells. Hence treatment-induced increases in naive CD4 and naive CD8 T cells were very modest compared to changes observed in rhGH-treated HIV patients. Additionally, despite anticipated negative effects of aging lymph nodes, positive results were seen. This study aims to prevent or reverse the typical age-related collapse of the TCR repertoire at ages just above those of our study population. As a result, the slight increases seen in these cells and in CD4 T-cell RTEs are compatible with this theory.

Epigenetic aging reversal may be accomplished via immunological and non-immunological processes. The particular combination of these drugs may activate a wide enough range of therapeutic pathways to explain the previously unpredictable reversal of epigenetic aging, even independently of the immunological markers we have measured. GH, DHEA, and metformin each have distinctive anti-aging effects.

In this regard, it is necessary to highlight the pro-aging properties of GH and IGF-1, which is why most gerontologists advocate lowering rather than raising these substances' levels. However, the use of mutations that influence the developmental programming of aging, which is not always applicable to nonmutant adults, confounds the majority of earlier investigations of aging and GH/IGF-1. For instance, these mutations in mice change the hypothalamus' normal innervation during brain development and stop hypothalamic inflammation in adults; hypothalamic inflammation may cause adults who are nonmutants to age throughout their bodies. Still, it is doubtful that reducing IGF-1 in healthy nonmutant adults will offer the same protection. The failure of previous Research to dissociate GH/IGF-1 signaling from changes in insulin signaling that occur throughout a lifetime is a second issue. Human longevity appears to be more consistently connected with insulin sensitivity than IGF-1 levels, which complicates the impact of IGF-1 on human longevity due to its inverse proportionality to insulin sensitivity. We feel that our approach of temporarily raising GH/IGF-1 while optimizing insulin sensitivity is justifiable in view of the good roles of GH and IGF-1 in immunological maintenance, the beneficial roles of immune maintenance in the prevention of aging, and our current findings.

Whatever the cause of the epigenetic age reversal may be, the four chosen epigenetic clocks all demonstrated a significant reduction in epigenetic age despite measuring aging in somewhat different ways and correlating with blood and leukocyte telomere length distinct ways. After 9 months of treatment, there was also a noticeable acceleration in the reversal of epigenetic aging. The latter observation's ramifications need more Research. Further, several epigenetic clocks that best predict human life expectancy and health span showed that epigenetic aging reversal appeared to partially return once therapy was stopped. This was

181

not the case for the grim Age clock. Whether subsequent assessments of epigenetic aging using the grim Age clock will reveal a consistent increase in expected life expectancy of two years or a gradual loss of improved life expectancy relative to baseline is still to be determined. In the latter case, it will be interesting to see if the trial therapy is repeated or extended to see if the expected longevity increase can be restored or increased.

Epigenetic age is the most precise indicator of biological age and the risk of developing age- related diseases currently available, although it does not account for all aspects of aging and not being the same as aging itself. This supports the use of epigenetic clocks to calculate the timeliness of estimates of the efficacy of potential anti-aging therapies. The current work demonstrates regression of epigenetic age with high statistical significance even in a one-year pilot trial including just 9 volunteers, providing strong support for this strategy. However, it will be necessary to replicate the current findings in a follow-up study with sufficient power to confirm them. Even if there is still much work to be done, the chances for a significant improvement in human aging seem extremely bright.

CHAPTER 23

FOUR EXPERIMENTAL TECHNIQUES

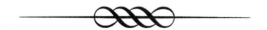

4.1 Finding and vetting volunteers

Following public disclosures of the trial's goals, ten ostensibly healthy adult men between the ages of 51 and 65 were recruited for the study by word-of-mouth. There were two cohorts, three men in the second and seven men in the first. Cohorts 1 and 2 received treatment from October 2015 to October 2016 and April 2016 to April 2017, respectively. Before providing a blood sample for objective validation of health eligibility, volunteers first completed an online screening questionnaire. Qualifying applicants then gave the sample. Candidates who passed the second screening were invited to a meeting for a physical examination, confirmation of their capacity to administer rhGH, baseline magnetic resonance imaging (MR) of the thymus, two additional blood draws (see Appendix S2), informed consent, and instructions on how to complete the provided medication diaries, which were designed to remind volunteers of their dosing schedules and to record any side effects or irregularities in dosing.

4.2.1 Trial procedure

The Aspire Institutional Review Board (Santee, California) approved the study protocol before the TRIIM trial's execution, and it was conducted under the supervision of IND 125,851 from the Food and Drug Administration. Under the supervision of the Stanford University Research Compliance Office, volunteers had MRI exams at the Lucas Center for Imaging, blood draws at the Stanford Blood Center, and CyTOF analyses at the Human Immune Monitoring Center (HIMC). The trial was carried out following the Declaration of Helsinki, the Obligations of Clinical Investigators, the Protection of Human Volunteers (21 CFR 50), and the Institutional Review Boards (21 CFR 56). (21 CFR 312). It was not preregistered on clinicaltrials.gov following FDA regulations for pre-Phase I exploratory studies (https://prsinfo.clinicaltrials.gov/ACT Checklist.pdf).

To get an initial insulin response, rhGH alone (0.015 mg/kg) was given during the first week of the trial. Then, during the second week, rhGH was mixed with 50 mg DHEA to test the effects of DHEA alone on insulin suppression. The same amounts of rhGH and DHEA were administered with 500 mg of metformin during the third week. All doses were tailored to the unique reactions of each volunteer beginning in the fourth week. After that, blood was taken a week before trial months 2, 3, 4, 6, and 9 to allow for additional dose changes at those periods (to optimize IGF-1 and decrease insulin), and more blood samples were taken after 12 months to wrap up the therapy monitoring period. The reaction of IGF-1, DHEAS, and insulin to the administration of rhGH, DHEA, and metformin, respectively, as well as regular communication with trial participants and a review of the medication diaries that were later returned, were used to confirm dosage compliance. For cohort 1, additional follow-up blood testing was performed at 18 months; cohort

2 was not accessible. In addition, supplemental blood collection was done at additional times in a few instances when it was deemed necessary.

Serum and peripheral blood mononuclear cells (PBMCs) were cryopreserved at the SBC, in the latter case using 10 percent dimethyl sulfoxide and fetal bovine serum, to permit simultaneous CyTOF analysis and further distribution of some samples to other centers (FBS). Until the trial's conclusion, these samples were kept there and then at the HIMC. To compensate for cell losses imposed by freezing and thawing or other reasons, Quest Diagnostics performed full blood counts. When presenting cell subsets as percentages of their reference populations (for example, naive CD4 cells as a percentage of all CD4 cells) and gating them to intact viable singlets, the requirement for adjustment was, however, typically avoided. Added blood tests are described in Appendix S2.

Trial participants received rhGH (Omnitrope, Sandoz), which they self-administered 3–4 times per week at bedtime along with other research drugs, depending on adverse effects.

Additionally, 3,000 IU of vitamin D3 and 50 mg of elemental zinc tablets were given to all volunteers and asked to be taken daily.

4.3 MR analysis and imaging

All imaging scans were performed at Stanford University's Lucas Center for Imaging using a single 3T GE Premier MRI scanner. Because there are no published standardized methods for quantitatively evaluating thymic fat content, we adopted a computational strategy that has previously been used to study the fat content of bone marrow (Hu, Nayak, & Goran, 2011). The thymic fat fraction (TFF) is measured using techniques that are more precise than a conventional histological examination by biopsy and range from 0% to 100%. (Fischer et al., 2012).

Three replicate core thymic zones were discovered in each examined time point as the fat-free thymic fraction (TFFF), which was computed as 100% - TFF. Additionally, the same methods were used to determine the sternal bone marrow fat-free fraction (BMFFF). For more details, see Appendix S2.

Immunophenotyping (4.4)

PBMCs that had been cryopreserved were thawed in a warm medium, twice washed, and then resuspended in CyFACS buffer (PBS supplemented with 2 percent BSA, 2 mM EDTA, and 0.1 percent sodiumazide). By excluding trypan blue dye, viability was assessed (Vi-CELL XR assay, Beckman Coulter Life Sciences). Next, 1.5 106 live cells were put on a V-bottom microtiter plate, and the cells were then washed once by being pelleted and resuspended in brand-new CyFACS solution. Finally, 50 l of a mixture of heavy metal isotope-labeled antibodies targeting 35 cell surface markers were used to stain the cells for 60 min on ice (for details and for details on cell washing, staining, permeabilization, and gating, see Appendix S2).

Establishing the epigenetic age

The degree of genomic DNA methylation in previously cry preserved PBMCs was evaluated by the Centre for Molecular Medicine and Therapeutics at the University of British Columbia.

Genomic DNA was isolated from tissues using the DNeasy Blood & Tissue Kit from Qiagen in Hilden, Germany. Genomic DNA was then methylated using the Zymo EZ DNA Methylation Kit (Zymo Research, Irvine, CA). Additionally, the Illumina Infinium Methylation EPIC Bead Chip (Illumina, San Diego, CA) was utilized to examine DNA methylation and measured single-CpG resolution DNAm levels at

866,836 CpG sites in the human genome (DNAm). This formula was used to quantify the amount of methylation at certain sites. Max(M,0) is the fluorescence intensity of methylated (M) alleles (signal A), and Max(U,0) is the fluorescence of unmethylated

(U) alleles (signal B). As a result, the range of values is 0 (completely unmethylated) to 1. (Dunning, Barbosa-Morais, Lynch, Tavare, & Ritchie, 2008).

To track worldwide trends in epigenetic aging, we first fit all-time point data to a linear mixed- effects model for longitudinal data (many types of blood drawn from the same person, corrected for the baseline DNAm age). From there, we computed the effects of the intervention on epigenetic age. Second, as described in the text, we calculated the change in epigenetic versus chronological age for each volunteer as (EA-A) - (EA-A)0, where EA is the epigenetic age at chronological age A and (EA-A)0 is the baseline difference between EA and A. This allowed us to isolate more precise individual- and time-specific changes.

Statistical investigation

To appropriately consider the information's longitudinal character, we used linear mixed-effects regression (multiple draws from the same person). In addition, we utilized standard linear or nonlinear regressions when adjusting for a time was not required. We used the t-test, the t-test for paired comparisons, or alternatives chosen by Sigma Plot where the assumptions underpinning t-tests were not supported for comparisons between pretreatment and specified post-treatment endpoints. Replicate findings for each volunteer at time zero were averaged, and each replicate result was split by the mean to provide a population of departures from 100 percent that could subsequently be utilized for comparison against later time points. This allowed for normalized comparisons to month

187

zero baselines. Independent hypothesis testing was typically not done, and in the case of both multiple tests for epigenetic age and significant differences in CyTOF results, all significant test results were highly correlated, making Bonferroni correction overly conservative. As a result, reported P values do not account for multiple comparisons.

MEANING OF WORDS USE

Heteroplasmy: is the presence of more than one type of organellar genome (mitochondrial DNA or plastid DNA) within a cell or individual. It is an important factor in considering the severity of mitochondrial diseases. Because most eukaryotic cells contain many hundreds of mitochondria with hundreds of copies of mitochondrial DNA, it is common for mutations to affect only some mitochondria, leaving most unaffected.

The suprachiasmatic nucleus or nuclei (SCN): is a tiny region of the brain in the hypothalamus, situated directly above the optic chiasm. It is responsible for controlling circadian rhythms. The neuronal and hormonal activities it generates regulate many different body functions in a 24-hour cycle. The mouse SCN contains approximately 20,000 neurons.

Cannabinoids: the word cannabinoid refers to every chemical substance, regardless of structure or origin, that joins the cannabinoid receptors of the body and brain and that have similar effects to those produced by the Cannabis Sativa plant.

PLEIOTROPY: refers to the phenomenon in which a single locus affects two or more apparently unrelated phenotypic traits and is often identified as a single mutation that affects two or more wild-type traits.

Monocytes: are a type of white blood cell (leukocytes) that reside in your blood and tissues to find and destroy germs (viruses, bacteria, fungi and protozoa) and eliminate infected cells. Monocytes call on other white blood cells to help treat injury and prevent infection.

Pluripotent stem cells: are cells that are able to self-renew by dividing and developing into the three primary groups of cells that make up a human body, including: Ectoderm: Giving rise to the skin and nervous system.

Methylation: is a chemical reaction in the body in which a small molecule called a methyl group gets added to DNA, proteins, or other molecules.

dehydroepiandrosterone

Dehydroepiandrosterone (DHEA) is a hormone that your body naturally produces in the adrenal gland. DHEA helps produce other hormones, including testosterone and estrogen. Natural DHEA levels peak in early adulthood and then slowly fall as you age.

hyperinsulinemia

Hyperinsulinemia means the amount of insulin in your blood is higher than what's considered normal

thixotropic

Thixotropy is a time-dependent shear thinning property. Certain gels or fluids that are thick or viscous under static conditions will flow (become thinner, less viscous) over time when shaken, agitated, shear-stressed, or otherwise stressed (time-dependent viscosity).

diabetogenic

A diabetogenic agent may be defined as one that produces a persistent elevation in blood-glucose concentration to within the values accepted by the Report of the International Expert Committee on the Diagnosis and Classification of Diabetes Mellitus

immunosenescence

Immunosenescence, defined as the changes in the immune system associated with age, has been gathering interest in the scientific and health-care sectors alike. The rise in its recognition is both pertinent and timely given the increasing average age and the corresponding failure to increase healthy life expectancy.

hyperhomocysteinemia

Hyperhomocysteinemia refers to the condition where there is greater than 15 micromol/L of homocysteine in the blood. This condition is present in a wide range of diseases, and in many cases, it is an independent risk factor for more serious medical conditions.

glucocorticoid

Glucocorticoids (GCs) are steroid hormones widely used for the treatment of inflammation, autoimmune diseases, and cancer. To exert their broad physiological and therapeutic effects, GCs bind to the GC receptor (GR) which belongs to the nuclear receptor superfamily of transcription factors.

hypomethylation

DNA hypomethylation refers to the loss of the methyl group in the 5-methylcytosine nucleotide. Methylation is a natural modification of DNA, and mainly affects the cytosine base (C) when it is followed by a guanosine (G) in mammals (Methylation).

Plasminogen

Plasminogen is an abundant plasma protein that exists in various zymogenic forms. Plasmin, the proteolytically active form of plasminogen, is known for its essential role in fibrinolysis.

cardiometabolic

Cardiometabolic diseases are a group of common but often preventable conditions including heart attack, stroke, diabetes, insulin resistance and non-alcoholic fatty liver disease. There is a global increase in the number of people who experience one or more of these conditions during their lifetime.

Insilico

InSilico offers a suite of technical indicators that gives traders access to raw market data visualized in ways that can help provide a deeper level of analysis, and help in making timely, informed trading decisions.

dinucleotide

a nucleotide consisting of two units each composed of a phosphate, a pentose, and a nitrogen base.

Printed in Great Britain
by Amazon